Watch Where You Point That Thing

Mastering Your Power of Intention

Lola Jones

This book is not intended to replace your own inner guidance,
nor to provide or replace medical advice.

Published by Lola Jones.
Printed in the United States of America.

ISBN: 978-0-9859026-1-2

Appreciation

Appreciation to the growing number of people who
share Divine Openings out of generosity and desire to contribute
to those they love, to the human race, and to the Universe itself.

Special appreciation goes to Russell Martin, who understands that I do my best to balance the solitary, internal life of a modern priestess with being a partner to him *and* a regular cowgirl. Besides being a brilliant author and filmmaker, Russell helps us with Divine Openings publishing, technical, and creative endeavors, and has organically become a part of all this. Thanks to all of you who contribute in the largest and smallest of ways. Appreciation for The Presence that created, empowers, enfolds, and Graces us all.

IMPORTANT NOTE:

To insure the high quality and purity of Divine Openings,

Lola Jones is currently the only person authorized

to initiate and certify Divine Openings Givers.

Table of Contents

Watch Where You Point That Thing

Introduction

Let there be light.
And there was light.

Let there be life.
And there was life.

Intend something, let go, and it happens.

Okay, that's all you need to know. End of book.

Seriously, this is true. Once you intend your desire, Life leads you there. So, why isn't this a one-page book? I asked that question and one more to my Large Self as I began to write: "What makes a person's power of intention stronger or weaker?" The Presence downloaded the answers over time.

While you'll explore a hundred profound new ways to raise your awareness and build your power of intention in the pages of this book, its two main themes are:

- How to get your limiting self out of the way, keep it out of the way, and let more good in, and,
- How to shift your identify toward your Large, unlimited Self.

Once you've done both, your power of intention soars. This book also offered me an opportunity to share, all in one place, many of the new downloads that have come since I wrote *Things Are Going Great In My Absence.*

As with all of Divine Openings, this is not work—I had a fantastic time writing this book and you'll enjoy feeling into it and putting it into practice. Two enormous regal red tail hawks are soaring together in circles just outside my window right now, always an auspicious sign that magic is happening.

Because Life *is* on our side, supports us, and brings everything we need, you may wonder why we would even need to *intend* or *ask* for anything? Why wouldn't we just relax, let The Divine decide what we need, and bring it to us?

Well, you *can* do that, and some people are content in that more passive role; but it's your birthright to be an active Co-Creator *with* The Presence, if you choose to be. From your perspective as a unique human, you know precisely what you'd like, because you're right in the thick of it in a physical body. The Presence appreciates your unique role in taking the Universe into new territories, new experiences, and new ideas that never existed before.

Using a business analogy, you're the human client telling the Universal supplier, your Large Self, what you want; the supplier is glad to know how to please you, and manufactures it. Good business people know that the client who's down there in the trenches daily darn well knows what he needs and wants, and that listening to the client is the best way to know what to produce on the client's behalf.

When I was a contract corporate trainer, I never offered canned programs, and companies appreciated that enormously. After first asking them about their needs, and learning what outcomes *they* wanted, I tailored

every single program to that client. I considered us co-creators of the experience rather than assuming I knew exactly what they needed or wanted, even though I was the expert in training and development. They were the ones doing the jobs and taking the risks.

You and The Presence are Co-Creators. The Presence cares to know what each unique physical human wants, and is the best listener you'll ever know—hearing, sensing, and feeling your intentions and desires *before* you ever speak them aloud.

Your wants and needs count. Your intentions are heard. Now—the only question is: how can you let it in more easily and fully?

With your intentions, fueled by your desires, you
participate actively in Creation.

If you just rolled along letting nature take its course like animals do, evolution would move more slowly, like it does in nature, where the stimulus for evolution is usually changes in environment or weather with a dollop of slow evolutionary impetus thrown in. Animals are not Conscious Creators like humans are. They don't say, "I wish I had a house instead of living in this hole." They'll live happily in a hole for millions of years. They don't say, "I wish I had a happier relationship with my spouse." When you add human consciousness, desire, and creativity to the mix, you get rapid evolution.

There are pros and cons to the way the animals live. Any animal is happier than most humans, because they are always in the Flow of Life. They accept "what is" without mental suffering because they have no logical mind to create suffering by judging right or wrong, good or bad. Their lives are simple.

But they are not Conscious Creators. Animals have simple desires, and they feel, react, and respond by instinct without suffering over whether they get those desires met. I do believe animals are evolving to be more conscious, some species rapidly, but that's another subject.

There are pros and cons to the way we humans live—we're not automatically in the Flow of Life— we can choose to be or not. We have *Free Will choices*. Humans have much more complex desires, which can make us unhappy or happy, depending on our attitude about our desires.

We humans actively shape our environment more than animals do. If an animal feels an ice age coming on, it adapts to the environment and grows a fuller fur coat and a thicker fat layer over several generations. If a human feels the climate getting colder, he doesn't grow more hair, he learns to make fire and make fur coats. Later, he builds shelters, invents indoor heating systems and warmer fabrics. Due to our unique gifts of *consciousness and creativity*, humans can now evolve dramatically in one lifetime. Humans are creators and rapid evolvers in a way that animals are not.

Human evolution wasn't always as fast as it is now. Not so long ago, humans believed it was the gods, nature, or their kings and priests who controlled their fates. Some humans are becoming aware of *how* we create, and as that power and responsibility is claimed, we become Conscious Creators, embodying The Presence, aware of itself, on Earth.

Prehistoric people around the globe used the same oval-shaped stone hand tool to skin animals and cut the meat for over a million years—that's almost zero evolutionary progress—very odd since their brains were growing larger. They made that tool instinctively, like birds build intricate nests. Then some Divine spark activated humanity, and a period of evolutionary momentum began. The changes were slow but speeded up steadily to today's exponential acceleration. There've been more revolutionary ideas and advances in just the last fifty years than in the past several thousand years, with stunning impact on our quality of life.

Whether you believe the Bible is a metaphor, a dusty, irrelevant text, or God's literal truth, my interpretation of the story of God telling Adam and Eve they would have dominion over all the other creatures in the Garden Of Eden is this: humans were given the power to create reality, and the animals were not. The humans would rule. The moment the humans ate the apple they began their journey to consciousness, beginning with a new *self-consciousness* of being naked. With the exception of dolphins and perhaps a few others, animals have no consciousness of themselves as beings, no awareness of what they look like, or what others think of them.

It's lovely to relax and allow your Large Self to guide you and bring you good things you wouldn't have ever thought of or believed possible. Allowing The Presence to bring new and wonderful things and experiences to you accelerates evolution if you just let go, get out of the way, and expand to make room to let it in. For years, I've just walked along letting Life lead me to things I only knew as vague inner longings.

It's also fun to ask for what you want and let The Presence cook it up for you. Sometimes you tell the chef to cook up his best dish for you, leaving the details to the kitchen, and other times you order exactly what you want—two eggs instead of three and toast instead of biscuits. This is the beauty and wonder of being human *and* Divine.

Find your own balance between intending your desires
and completely letting go to the Flow Of Life.

The question, "My will or God's will?" just isn't useful—it just separates you from your Large Self. When you're being your Large Self, there is no difference between your will and God's. There is a useful distinction between your small self's will and your Large Self's will up to a point in your evolution, but once you live life as your Large Self most of the time there really is no distinction between your will and God's. You'll outgrow the Large Self/small self labels I introduced in *Things Are Going Great In My Absence*. In the meantime, please, please do not make your small self wrong or bad. That just won't serve you.

If you get upset at the difficult lives some humans have, consider that they're not yet Conscious Creators. They're creating their reality *unconsciously* every day, unaware of *how* they're doing it. Now that you are a Conscious Creator, your life has infinite possibilities, but you cannot directly create for other humans, you can only add your enlightenment to the collective, indirectly helping it evolve. Even though on the largest level, you are they, and they are you, you are living individualized lives, making different choices. You can demonstrate how to be conscious and offer your love and help—they can accept or decline. Don't worry too much if you can't help someone; life is eternal, and The Presence, who's living all of it as all of us, isn't worried.

Most of you look back on your life before reading *Things Are Going Great In My Absence* and see it as your shift from *unconscious creator* or *partially conscious creator* to *Conscious Creator*. Everything you created before your awakening feels like a different life—and you have a new, more expanded life now.

In a most wonderful way, you were let off the hook for the past—you could write it off because *you didn't know* back then—but you take responsibility now and going forward. You didn't have to fix all your issues from childhood and your past; the old issues, problems, and limits began to fade away as you moved into this newly enlightened consciousness and started living from today. You replaced the old reality rather than trying to fix it.

Each year my own words in *Things Are Going Great In My Absence,* which I wrote six years ago, get clearer and mean more to me. Reading it still gives me new elevations. Divine Openings is living, evolving Energy, Light, and Intelligence, not a dead text or a set dogma. These books are alive in the most real sense.

People ask me all the time, "How did you get that powerful energy into the art in your book?"

"I intended it," I answer.

"How do you create a field of resonance that changes lives?"

"I intend it."

I have no method, so intending it is all there is to it! But this points up the truth that just knowing something isn't enough. You could read a medical surgery text, but could you perform a surgery?

To put a lighter spin on this, one of my fitness gurus, Tony Horton, says on his fun DVDs, "you got to bring it!" In *Jerry Maguire*, Tom Cruise shouted, "Show me the money!" Going even farther back, remember the Wendy's ad with the little old lady demanding, "Where's the beef?" That became popular slang for "Where's the real substance, the meat of the matter?"

Ha! There's a setup for you. The Presence just said, "The meat of *this* matter isn't *matter.* It's not physical matter—it's Non-Physical." The Presence is such a cut-up.

I capitalize Non-Physical throughout this book to emphasize its importance, because increasing your focus on the Non-Physical builds your power enormously, yet it's admittedly challenging to focus on something you can't see, hear, or feel most of the time. *Things Are Going Great In My Absence* heightens your Non-Physical awareness and experience, and this book takes you much deeper into the Non-Physical.

In the Non-Physical there is no work, so the minute you start "working on *yourself*" or "working on *it*" you're back in physical focus, in the old paradigm. Your power is in the Larger Non-Physical aspect of your being. Power of intention reduces your dependence on the physical, and you stop trying to fix, shine up, or manipulate the physical. There's already enough work in the physical realm—oh, you've already noticed that!

If you haven't already, you must drop the "I have *issues* to resolve" belief. Leave that back there in the old paradigm, too. As your more limited self, you could spend your life trying to push rocks up hills in the physical realm, or you could just move deeper into living as your unlimited Large Self, which has no "issues" and no rocks to push. None!

Intend to embark on this adventure light, free, and playful, no matter how serious or urgent you imagine your needs and blocks to be. The Presence doesn't see any blocks, and none of it is serious, difficult, or impossible at all. Agree with The Presence—that's a good start!

Leave the "working on it" and "issues" paradigm behind.

Take a moment to reboot and refresh your understanding of the word *vibrate*, because we're going to use it a lot. One reason I made up a lot of new terms in Divine Openings is that sometimes we hear a word so many times we can't really hear it anymore. If your mind stuffs an important idea into a box that's too small for it, or distorts it to make it fit an old paradigm, it loses its power and effectiveness *instantly*.

So here's a fresh way to perceive *vibration* as we'll use it here. You've seen animations where a cartoon broadcast tower pulses radial waves outward from it. The sound is "ping, ping, ping, ping" as it steadily pulses its message. That is what you are, a broadcast tower, pulsing out invisible Non-Physical signals powerful enough to reach across the globe and beyond the Universe to all dimensions. These Non-Physical signals pull people, things, and circumstances to you that match up with the frequencies you pulse. Other beings feel and read the pulses and are either drawn or repelled.

Under a microscope you can actually see living cells pulsing with life. Your entire being, down to the cells, molecules, and atoms, dances to a rhythm that varies as you focus on different subjects. As you think about a happy area of your life your energy field may be dancing to a light tune, "ping, ping, ping," but as you think about a not-so-happy area of life it slows down to a heavy funeral march, "bhloooonnnph, bhloooonnnph, bhloooonnnph."

For example: as a woman thinks about the work she loves, her tower pulses out ping, ping, ping, bright and high-frequency, high on the Instrument Panel, because she feels the same as her Large Self does in that department. But as her thoughts drift to her relationship with her daughter, the pulses are dull and at a slower and lower frequency, quite apart from how her Large Self experiences it, so she doesn't feel good.

If she's allowing and appreciating those lower feelings, they give her a valuable Instrument Panel reading, cueing her to adjust to pulse more in agreement with her Large Self's high, steady ping— then she feels good. As pulses emit from her, Life sends matching physical-world components to meet them. Her work is already joyful and successful, and once she adjusts her broadcast about her daughter, they get along better.

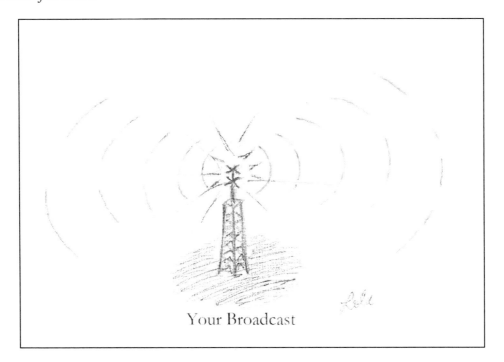

Your Broadcast

This book guides you through experiences that expand and prepare you until you're not just thinking your intentions, you're literally pulsing them, broadcasting them like a giant radio tower. At that point, creating by intention becomes incredibly easy.

Working at it doesn't help—relaxing helps. Thinking hard or figuring it out doesn't help—feeling more helps. Being smart doesn't help—letting go helps. The only thing I'm mule-stubborn about is being powerful and keeping my vibration up. I will not let go of that! No way!

Relax, and take the ride.

This is a good time to stop and assimilate these first pages. Your mind may be saying, "I got it," or "I already knew that," but there's more happening here than just transfer of intellectual knowledge—it's more than the mind knows.

Frequent assimilation is vital. I had to stop and assimilate as I wrote this book—it gave me indigestion to write as fast as I usually do. This was entirely new for me. That didn't happen even when I was writing the powerful self-paced online retreat Jumping The Matrix. Our precious human body can't always run at the speed of spirit.

When you see these asterisks, stop and breathe consciously. Feel the oxygen travel throughout your body, and savor how good that feels. Feel this vibration energizing your cells with pure power of intention. Feel and embrace anything that arises.

* * * * * * * *

Build On A Solid Foundation

This book isn't intended to stand alone—it builds upon a foundation established in my previous book *Things Are Going Great In My Absence: How To Let Go And Let The Divine Do The Heavy Lifting.* The Energy / Light / Intelligence and the Divine Openings in *Things Are Going Great In My Absence* initiate your enlightenment, expand your pipes, and tune you in to higher frequencies. This book assumes all of that has already happened. If you want to master calculus (this book), get the foundational math and geometry first (*Things Are Going Great).*

If you're building a house, lay the foundation and let it cure before you build on it. *Things Are Going Great In My Absence* is a solid foundation of a *specific type* that we haven't seen anywhere else. *Things Are Going Great In My Absence* teaches you to read your Instrument Panel, brings you to a place of genuine appreciation for those feelings and events you used to call problematic, and accelerates your evolutionary pace. It walks you through experiences this book does not repeat.

The experiential foundation *Things Are Going Great In My Absence* provides cannot be duplicated, skipped, or summarized. Read it again if you haven't actually done all of the practical exercises. It's easy to order *Things Are Going Great In My Absence* at www.DivineOpenings.com/books.

Because *Things Are Going Great In My Absence*, initiated people into enlightenment, you might wonder why there would be any need for another book at all. For some people, there isn't a need, but because everyone is different, people are in widely varying degrees of mastery after reading *Things Are Going Great In My Absence.*

The awakening is gradual for most people (but not all.) Even those who don't *need* additional support still enjoy focusing on things that match and support their new reality, as much of the world *does not* support it. My goal is to provide fun, productive ways to focus, expand, and enjoy that don't take you backward into seeking, processing, and working on issues.

Divine Openings always takes you deeper into yourself.

Everyone lets go at different rates, so some people need more assistance or more time. Some doggedly hold onto old, long-practiced resistances or comfort zones longer than others. We humans, including me, like to do it "our way," and even if it isn't working, we often stubbornly resist—until the day we let go. One woman told me she resisted Divine Openings for two years, looking for any loophole to avoid feeling, before she finally let go and stepped into a whole new freedom.

Different aspects of us wake up at different times. As your consciousness expands, you'll be able to hear more each time you read this. Each time, you'll apply it to the changing circumstances in your life.

Read each book slowly, and several times.

There's a stair-step effect. You elevate, and from that level you can see more possibilities and claim more power, which you then use to go even higher. You keep leap-frogging yourself upward. This is the ever-expanding nature of the enlightened life—evolution through joy, momentum, and intention more than through pain, failure, problems, suffering, and struggle.

Experience takes you to practical mastery, far beyond analyzing, theorizing, talking, and reading about it. You must experience something to truly own it, and some people must experience it a number of times to own it and live into it. Experience has always been Divine Openings' strength—this is where the rubber meets the road.

To truly own it, experience it.

Here's a piece of timeless spiritual wisdom: "Love everyone." It's easy to say it, but to carry it out requires practical mastery. We all know love is the answer. Can everyone live it? Knowing something and living it are two different things.

I'm not content to merely pass along knowledge, even cutting-edge knowledge. Divine Openings offers experience and vibrational adjustments. You're getting one right now even as we ramp up.

We all have our areas of genius. Mine is Divine Openings. I'm a specialist in translating raw new leading-edge energies into practical, useable form for others. Gifted experts who have developed their specialized areas of expertise are a blessing to us all; I don't want to do my own software design—I just want to *use* and benefit from leading-edge technology. Their innovations—Internet, software, hardware, services, and apps—make what I do possible. I call the vet, the electrician, or the plumber to help me with things I just have no aptitude for. Accordingly, some people turn to teachers or physical healers for specialized insights, maintenance, and training.

Let me put it plainly: you have practical mastery of *Things Are Going Great In My Absence* when you are generally no longer suffering. Your life is not perfect; you are still expanding and evolving; you still have some challenges and lower vibrations about certain subjects, but you're not suffering over it. You are enjoying the ride, navigating, savoring the waiting, surfing your feelings, and embracing and valuing them all. That's when you're positioned to get the most of what this book offers.

Things Are Going Great In My Absence activated and awakened you *to* the Large Self that's in you and encompasses you. From that place, this book can yield more of the secret, hidden treasure inside of you, and even more evidence that you are in complete control of your personal reality.

You're making it all up.
The only question is, are you enjoying what you're making up?

Experience this book with an empty mind that has open space in it. Whenever you see the asterisks, stop and breathe consciously. Feel the oxygen travel throughout your body, blank your mind, dive in and assimilate.

* * * * * * * *

Enjoy Evolving Over Time

For five years, I didn't even think about writing a book to follow *Things Are Going Great In My Absence*. Readers who committed to using the material and giving up seeking were doing fabulously. I'm unable to stop creating, and all my new material was being poured into online courses and retreats because I so enjoy the multimedia and the flexibility to update and change them as this fast-moving consciousness evolves. I was having fun writing my humor book, *Confessions Of A Cowgirl Guru,* making music, painting, leading Five Day Silent Retreats, and taking much needed time to balance out with a richer, more satisfying personal life.

Author friends would ask me, "When's your next book coming out?" and I'd joke, "We don't need another book—that one did it." That book, the online courses, and the live retreats take many, many people to a place of mastery, automatic evolution, and ongoing expansion without working on themselves. I let this book percolate, knowing it would emerge in good time. Once that happened, I could not stop writing.

And here it is.

Reading the book *Things Are Going Great In My Absence* and doing the optional Self-Paced Level One Online Retreat get people beyond suffering, and help them attain some appreciation of emotions and mastery of the Instrument Panel, freeing up energy to go even higher.

Feeling *pain* is one of the many contrasts of human life, and is valuable information, but if you find yourself *suffering* for longer than a day or two *about anything*, go back and actively experience *Things Are Going Great*, take Level One Online Self-Paced, and listen to the audios of me teaching and counseling. It will be just as if I am talking to you. If you've lived something a long time, it can be a blind spot for you, where I can see it clearly.

Pain + resisting the experience = suffering.

If you're still suffering, perhaps you just *read* the experiential parts of Level One instead of *doing them*—mere reading doesn't bring practical mastery. Also, each time you read *Things Are Going Great,* your consciousness expands, so, on your next reading you hear things you just couldn't hear before. People ask me if I sneaked in while they were sleeping and added new material to *Things Are Going Great* since they last read it.

I know someone is really getting it when they write me: "I used to be in a big hurry to get to Jumping The Matrix (Level Three Online.) Now I'm enjoying the ride so much I don't want Level Two (which is all about living in joy) to end, so I've slowed down, hoping to extend the enjoyment of the Level Two course for another year!"

Yes! That's it!

Slower is faster with Divine Openings. Paradoxically, people tell me the good in their lives accelerates *faster* when joy is the goal, not working on themselves or attaining some imagined state of perfection.

The exhilaration of the wind blowing your hair back is the point,
not your speed, or reaching a destination.

Watch Where You Point That Thing is specifically focused on *building your power of intention.* Its web companion, the Self-Paced Level Two Online Retreat, has a broader scope and includes even more new topics than this book, plus, you get audios and videos you can stream or download. Activities and meditations from this book, recorded in my voice, help you bring it down to Earth and apply it in your life.

This book and Level Two Online are about your new life beyond suffering, working on yourself, and tedious processing. It's about enjoying the thrill of expansion, becoming a powerful Conscious Creator—that is who you *are.*

Each time I write a new book or online program it stretches *me* and requires that I undergo evolution. That's the fun of eternal expansion. As I download the words and energies from the Non-Physical, I must get up to speed with it myself before I can express the clearest vibrational essence of it. Otherwise, it's mere words, and I'm far too result-oriented to mess around with that.

If you haven't already, you'll soon come to enjoy eternal expansion for its own sake, with no need to get anywhere. It's lovely to be happy with now, knowing more is coming—without needing to make it happen or fix anything. Just stay relaxed, awake, and aware, and life rockets along.

Slower is often faster.

Here's why life accelerates when you let go. The Presence considers you perfect in your imperfection—always—right now. When you make who or where you are wrong, you take yourself instantly out of alignment with The Presence. You are clinging to the "something needs fixing" rock in the rapids and get battered instead of letting go to the Flow of Life. When you release resistance and let go of the rock, the Flow Of Life sweeps you along easily.

As soon as you relax and truly feel the perfection of this moment throughout your entire being, you are restored to full agreement with The All That Is, and can recognize and let in the good that is always being offered to you.

You are right now at the verge of an accelerated journey, yet how fast you "get there" isn't the point. You want to expand and experience what's next, and next, and next, and you have eternity to enjoy that. Watch birds in the sky flying for the joy of it, and get ready to spread your wings and soar— eternally. Of course you'll get impatient at times. Just smile and breathe.

For now, focus first on *how you want to feel* rather than on material manifestations you think will *give you that feeling,* no matter how urgent your needs are. Savor each moment. You'll be amazed at what happens.

Life accelerates when you embrace now, yet keep moving.

In *Things Are Going Great In My Absence,* you received Divine Openings by gazing at the art works, although many of you could feel the Divine Openings while reading or even holding the book—the intention of that book was that clear and powerful.

In keeping with this book's increased focus on the all-encompassing Non-Physical realm, there is a huge Non-Physical component to this book—you're getting far more than words and concepts. I've intended much Non-Physical assistance for you.

It's not like *Things Are Going Great In My Absence,* however, because you had enlightenment initiations in that book, and an evolutionary acceleration occurred. There are no Divine Openings in this book. Instead of amping the energy up more, you'll ground those energies more into the physical realm, and move to the next level of bringing your desires down to Earth.

With Divine Openings, and the energies that are already coming to us, you don't need more energy; you need to ground what you're already getting. If you ever feel a sense of tension, like you're revved up more than you can handle, you need to ground that energy in your physical body. It's as if you're pushing the accelerator, or the evolutionary forces are pushing on your accelerator, but your other foot is on the brake. The brake represents resistance to letting go to the energy you already have or allowing yourself to move as you're being called to move.

You probably don't need more acceleration—I'll remind you of this more than once. You need to assimilate, get your foot off the brake, and relax so Grace can carry you. This book is designed for that.

Don't ask for more energy—ask to let go to what you already have.

When you resist the new energies, or resist letting in what you truly want, it's supposed to hurt, so you'll move.

This book does help you ground the new frequencies now available to facilitate our evolution, expansion, and power of intention. Our planet is virtually being bombarded with new energies—if you're resisting, it feels like pressure—if you're not resisting, it feels like bliss.

There is no processing—there's nothing for you to do once you master this except stay awake, play with it, and enjoy. Each section deepens your ability, and typically:

- Helps you let go of what you're not in control of.
- Helps you get out of the way.
- Gives you something fun or productive to feel and do with what you *are* in control of.
- Helps you live as your Large Self more of the time.

You need not memorize, analyze, or figure anything out, but simply enjoy. How fantastic is that?

Intend to assimilate, enjoy, and ground it as you go.

In the rest breaks at the end of each section, intend to align with and assimilate that section. Enjoy the breaks like a treat or mini-vacation, and let The Divine do the heavy lifting.

Here's an assimilation break:
Stop and breathe consciously. Feel the delicious oxygen travel to every cell in your body. Close your eyes, go deep within, blank your mind as much as you can. Let The Presence assimilate this into your body at a deeper level, beyond the mind. If your mind interferes, let that drift on by and refocus. Each time you refocus you will go deeper.

* * * * * * * *

Claiming Your Own Power

Enjoy living into this book. Be deliberately, intentionally conscious about it, and with eyes wide open, notice what happens, and Life will give you all the feedback you need to get better at it. If what you're doing is not working, you can change it rather than arguing with Life.

I've proven the methods in this book to myself, both by doing them and having them work, and by not doing them and suffering the consequences! Yes, I too sometimes crazily, stubbornly try to buck the laws of the Universe and get things to work *my way.* But it gets tiring, it feels awful, and I give it up as soon as I can. Whether something works or doesn't work, we gain clarity either way.

Effectiveness is the measure of truth.

No matter how smart you are, slow down—savor each sentence, tasting it, feeling it, experiencing it in your practical life's daily context. Experience brings it down to Earth in your life. Make a game of seeing how long you can make this book last.

One woman wrote that she couldn't read more than a sentence or two of *Things Are Going Great In My Absence* at a time, because it set off explosions of feeling and knowing in her that demanded she stop—and each time she stopped, it took her on a deep inner journey. Mere reading causes you to miss what only experience can provide.

Some humans have an unconscious drive to give their power to an authority figure who promises to relieve them from having to *experience,* feel, think, take risks, make their own choices, and learn to read their own Instrument Panel. Yes, even after reading *Things Are Going Great In My Absence,* a few still want to give their power away. I mention this *again* because seeking addiction is so commonplace in the metaphysical world that people can get mired in it without noticing or fall back into it after getting free. What you want is within you, and Divine Openings always guides you deeper within.

If you want mastery, make a commitment not to dilute this with other books, seminars, sessions, and modalities for at least one year. Incompatible modalities are those that have you work on yourself, have others work on you, introduce other energies, or promise to fix your emotions for you. Acupuncture and chiropractic are compatible, because they don't introduce energies; they open and balance your own. Bodywork with no energy work in it helps you relax, and thereby release resistance.

As I pointed out in *Things Are Going Great In My Absence*, with Divine Openings you can make modalities, teachers, or things with zero power appear to help you—but you *gave* them the power to do that—*your power*. Things can get very confusing from there; you can drift away from Divine Openings, which is all about going within, and after a while those other things stop working because they had no power in the first place, and now you have given all your power away and are back to seeking and struggling, wondering, "What happened?"

People who mix energies and modalities, work on themselves, and have others work on them are the most confused and disempowered people we encounter. If they're willing, we keep steering them back to their own inner power.

In the Level Two Online Retreat, there's a great audio called *Stay Awake, Own Your Power*, a session with a woman who gave her power to a teacher, but was called back to consciousness by her Large Self.

Divine Openings continually, steadily points you
within, to your own power.

Each time I write a course or book, it's such a pleasure to see that the synchronicities were building up to it for decades! When I was a contract trainer leading courses in people skills and management at corporations, the participants would quickly begin to talk about feeling enlightened, and I *never said those words*—in fact I carefully avoided spiritual language and used only business terms, but my powerful intention prevailed, communicated vibrationally, and the Non-Physical message was received anyway.

My subtext—the words not said under the main text, was always enlightenment—and the intention played out for all who were ready and willing to let it in. That is the power of intention.

As an interesting aside, I created the terms Large Self and small self around 1993 to use in those corporate settings because they are neutral and universal, not spiritual. I could sketchily introduce the idea of Large Self and small self and everyone innately knew what I was talking about, and they would describe the qualities of Large and small self while I merely recorded them on the flip chart. Those terms tapped into some universal truth in everyone.

From engineers at IBM to workers at a plant, not a single person ever resisted it; they recognized these disparate elements of themselves, and this let them identify them, become more conscious of them, and begin to choose their own state more deliberately. That told me something Larger was already accessible to every human being, and simply focusing on it initiated an awakening to that more expanded aspect of who they were.

Many of them had never given a thought to anything beyond the physical world, or had been turned off by religious dogma or spiritual airy-fairy stuff.

Luxuriate in this lush vibratory field that we've created for you in this book. Let in the magic of the intention embedded in the book. The vibration of it assists you to activate your power—the power that's already within you. One thing is certain: you'll have to ignore what most of the world is doing, and how they're doing it. You'll be a bit of a renegade. An evolutionary revolutionary.

The back of my business card says:

Evolutionary
Author
Teacher
Artist
Singer
Songwriter
Cowgirl

Be an evolutionary revolutionary.

Your Large Self is hugely expansive and indefinable. Intend to let go of all your self-definitions and self-limitations so you can expand beyond them—they are not really you. Let go of all you know so you can know more.

The best news in this book is that we don't have to be perfect, because Life and Grace are on our side. If we can just keep ourselves reasonably clear, Grace tips the balance for us. Support from Non-Physical is so incredibly powerful that we can't mess it up no matter what we do. We can create temporary challenges for ourselves, but there is never, ever any permanent damage.

Take a deep breath and relax into the support that is there for all of us. We can let go, do the best we can, and enjoy the ride.

* * * * * * * *

How To Build Your Power Of Intention
Or: Here's The Beef

You've done step one. Reading *Things Are Going Great In My Absence* prepared you for this book by initiating your enlightenment, giving you your Level One foundation in the conscious mind piece, and giving you appreciation of your Instrument Panel. And all along you thought you were just feeling better, but that was more important than you could possibly imagine at the time.

Feeling better becomes your springboard into a fabulous new reality because feeling better clearly indicates you've reached a higher vibration. It's very hard to get where you want to go from *not* feeling good about it, and much easier when you're vibrating higher on that subject. You don't have to be perfect now or ever—just a slight upward trajectory will do just fine.

Thoughts, feelings, and vibration are bridges to
your Non-Physical power.

The most important factor in my power of intention is that I'm passionately devoted to feeling good and maintaining as high a vibrational state in every moment as I can. It feels bad to me to stray from it, and you know by now: straying from your Large Self's perspective is *supposed to feel bad.*

Ponder these questions and let the answers emerge from within you as we go. Later on, you're going to find that the following questions are an especially powerful type of question. Just saying them to yourself plants seeds that will yield results:

> What's going on with people who have big "power of intention"?

> How can they just say it or think it and it appears?

> What are they doing, and not doing?

> How can I become one of those Creators who can just "dial it in?"

What makes the difference? Obviously, it's not just having more esoteric knowledge. I'll guide you more by vibrational attunement and feeling than by thinking. Beyond words, this book gives you experiences that grow your power of intention.

You'll notice your power of intention increasing.

ACTIVITY: The Black and White Meditation

This meditation is wonderful for those whose minds are busy and difficult to still. Close your eyes, smile gently, and imagine you're sitting in a movie theater with a black movie screen in front of you. Then, it becomes a brightly-lit white screen before it becomes black again. Breathe in on the white screen, and out on the black screen, back and forth at your own pace. Breathe in this way for five minutes, and then slowly open your eyes. Stretch and savor how you feel.

Level Two Online contains an audio that guides you through this activity, with my original music in the background.

Consciously merging with your Large Self feels delicious.
It's pleasure—not work.

* * * * * * * *

The World Is Becoming More Non-Physical

It's endlessly amusing to me that so much of our physical world is becoming more Non-Physically focused and less physically manifest as we rocket into this exponentially accelerated stage of evolution. The cosmic joke is that work, entertainment, media, communication, commerce, money—so much of it is becoming more and more Non-Physical.

The Internet is Non-Physical! If you think about it, a website doesn't really have *form* in the way we used to think about physical form. Our online courses exist only in cyberspace. There's no weight or mass to any of them. And when I've looked inside the silver box that's my Mac laptop, my website isn't in there. Neither are my photos, movies, books, or songs. All I've seen were some circuit boards, wires, metal, and chips with some data somehow stored on them. Fortunately, it all translates to sounds, colors, words, and shapes that make sense to us.

One day, I realized that the massive content of my enormous website is basically Non-Physical. My Non-Physical Large Self inspired me to have the mental thoughts to pour onto the keyboard, then my computer converted them into energy and code, then your computer translated them to look like a website. It's really just electrons bouncing around in cyberspace. There's nothing there.

Our audios are mostly downloads that are silent bits of code that only become sound waves when you play them. People's music is mostly on iPods now instead of physical CDs. All this stuff barely exists!

The waves that send television, radio, microwave, and cell phone signals to us are invisible and soundless. Your television, radio, stereo, or phone reads the signals and turns them into colorful pictures and sounds! The information flies through the air on waves and somehow doesn't get mixed up with other waves. If we could see all the waves and vibrations in the air around us it would be wondrous indeed.

Most of the information you need in your world is probably stored on a computer or accessed on the Internet. I take my Mac on a trip and have everything I use in my work with me: handouts, music, slide shows, photographs, movie editing, sound recording, email, and the ability to edit my website via the Internet. I used to have several file cabinets in my office, and now I have two small drawers of files, and one box of tax records in the garage that I'll never look at again.

After the Five Day Silent Retreat, people don't take home anything physical, yet people leave with transformed lives. They don't need anything material, but for later support I do give them access to a special online area for further training and development. And it's not physical either!

More and more people are reading books on Kindles and iPads rather than physical books. We take all this for granted so much that it wakes us up just to focus on it.

We knock on a table, and it is solid. What is it really? It's energy vibrating. Our eyes, ears, and other senses perceive it as solid, impenetrable, and heavy, although scientists assure us it's mostly space. They can barely find any *physical* there!

We think money is physical, but actually, money is very Non-Physical and abstract, and becoming more so every day. Money is now mostly plastic cards that cause ones and zeroes to appear and disappear on a super-computer. Your bank account is numbers on a computer. Your debt, if you have any, consists of numbers on a computer. Your mortgage is mostly numbers on a computer.

The stock market is mostly *perceived value* and numbers on a computer. More and more people get paperless bills and pay each other online.

Money has become a cosmic joke, so laugh along,
realize how unreal it is, and you'll lighten up about it.

I'm starting to rave with appreciation about this, and just pointing my attention at it thrills me and fills me with possibility. It's magical and enchanting. Technology has leveled the playing field to allow any person to wield the power that used to be reserved for large organizations with many employees. Internet sites now have the reach and the audiences once reserved only for television networks. Musicians can get heard on YouTube.

Of course, old forms, structures, and jobs disappear. That has always happened. There are no more horse drawn buggy manufacturers—those people moved to jobs in the auto industry. Today, fewer people are making physical things—they're offering Non-Physical services.

You can focus on your power or bemoan the lack of it, and either way you will be right. Your attention inadvertently becomes intention.

Attention becomes intention.
Watch where you point that thing.

A major key to building your power of intention is to nurture a steady awareness that this bag of flesh and bone, while wonderful, is not all there is of you—it's only a small part of your arsenal of resources. That's the Larger Perspective that informs my life and provides power and peace at the same time. *Intend now* to let this become a deeper and more tangibly powerful knowing for you rather than an ineffectual, dry intellectual concept.

I had occasion to observe a surgery just a couple of feet away from the operating table, suited up in scrubs, looking over the surgeons' shoulders while they opened the skull of a three-year-old child to reconstruct her severely deformed head and face. Undisturbed as they literally peeled her face off her skull to roll it out of the way, I was fascinated and quietly aware that the child's body was merely a small part of the totality of who she was, and I felt her as a powerful being, not limited to that small body. I celebrated with her Large Self while her human self lay there unconscious. They were working on her mechanically, but she was so much more than that mechanical body.

Whenever you find a physical reality too distracting, stop and focus within, remembering who you are. Who you are is far Larger, vaster, and more enduring than your current physical body, your current physical situation, and your current emotional state. Your physical body is temporary, your emotions are ephemeral, and your entire current reality is but the blink of any eye in eternity.

Knowing at deeper and deeper levels of your being that physical, temporary realities are fleeting, you relax about current reality, and without resistance to it, it morphs and shifts more easily. Whenever a current situation isn't pleasing to me, my habit is to say to myself, "It's temporary." And so it is.

It's all temporary.

Because what you focus on is expanded and energized by your attention, stay awake and be aware of what you choose to give your powerful attention to. Not choosing is still choosing: it's taking the default choice and letting somebody else, or circumstances, determine what you focus on.

Focus on the Non-Physical. I'll give you powerful ways to practice this nebulous task of focusing on essentially Nothing! It gets easier. As you focus more on the Non-Physical, it becomes more and more fundamentally real to you. Soon, the Non-Physical is more real to you than the physical, and you'll prove it to yourself over and over. Life gets much lighter when you truly understand that it's actually comprised of Nothing.

Focus deliberately.

Many of you could read only a few pages of *Things Are Going Great In My Absence* at a time before you fell into a deep sleep. There is great value in that, as you assimilate best when you're "out of the way." Please read a little bit, then take long, leisurely breaks in between sections or even paragraphs, to stare empty-headed out the window, take a walk, or enjoy a luscious nap. This allows for integration of the new vibration, and gives it space to deepen, expand, and take hold before you move on.

The mind can be speedy and greedy if you've trained it to engulf books and modalities without fully experiencing them.

It's the empty spaces between the notes that give beauty and richness to the song, while providing contrast and relief for the ear. The empty spaces between your thoughts give richness and contrast to your life, and give the brain a chance to rest and digest. Gorging just gives you indigestion.

Rest and assimilate.

* * * * * * * *

Beyond Spiritual

As I've evolved, the word "spiritual" feels less and less relevant and more and more limiting and artificial to me—as if there's some special department of life called spiritual, and another mundane department called the physical world, and that they're separate somehow. The mind loves to separate, divide, label, and analyze. That works great for some things, but not for other things like love, joy, relationships, and pure creation.

Beginning when I was a child, it made no sense to me how God and regular life were somehow split apart. God was up there. We were down here. God seemed to be too busy to pay any attention to our daily lives, and we were too busy doing what had to be done to pay much attention to God. We didn't know the Non-Physical was accessible right here—we thought Heaven was separate from the physical, only to be experienced after death.

Spirituality and religion were intangible, and the physical world felt more real. The physical world certainly is intense and in our face, demanding our moment-to-moment attention.

With the thousands of diverse definitions, there's a lot of baggage attached to the word spiritual, just as there is with the word God. It's hard to untangle spirituality from dogma and stereotypes of what spirituality is or "should be." If you have baggage about the word spiritual, I suggest you ditch it and focus on the Non-Physical, freeing you to have a fresh, authentic, direct experience.

Speaking of baggage, I must share a joke The Presence woke me with today: If Divine Openings was an airline, we'd be called Air Freedom. Our motto and pledge to our customers: "Give us your baggage with confidence. We promise, we *WILL* lose it!"

The Non-Physical is now more real and potent to me than this physical world. I know in my bones, beyond my mind's ability to explain it, that physical is transient, and Non-Physical is real and eternal—that the Non-Physical aspect of ourselves is vastly more powerful than our physical selves. It is the steady, enduring Source where our temporary physical selves originate.

I don't say that to diminish or devalue our precious physical selves, but to put it into perspective. It's vital for us to recognize that the physical selves we focus into this physical plane are but a tiny fraction of our Larger, Non-Physical selves.

Your Non-Physical Self can't be fully contained in your physical body. There is incomprehensibly more of *you* in the Non-Physical than there is of you here in the physical. Life is broadened and we are immensely empowered by expanding our awareness of who and what we are beyond the physical confines of our bodies. Just intend to experience this, and it expands you.

Life is all one flow. There's no need to break it down into separate departments, designating some things, activities, substances, and places as spiritual, sacred, mundane, or profane. That makes no sense in my reality. I don't go to church—it seems absurd, like having to go to a certain building each week to love my lover or to learn new things. I don't attend spiritual activities or groups because I don't need support. I generate support for myself, and draw it from within. Life is full of that all-permeating vibration, Energy, Love, Grace, and Intelligence. All is God.

I AM that vibration—yes, even when I'm not being "good." There's nowhere to go to find it, and I can't lose it anyway. How satisfying it is to live that most of the time.

The Non-Physical is the great force behind the physical world we experience with our human senses. The Non-Physical is the Larger, eternal, expanded, unlimited power that gives birth to our physical world. It keeps your heart beating, your lungs pumping, your liver filtering, and your body animated.

You don't have to know how it works to tap into it every day.

The Non-Physical is infinite, encompassing, ineffable, indefinable, and mysterious, yet it is accessible to you. All the fleeting manifestations of the physical world emerge from and return to the Non-Physical. In this book we move deeper into your Non-Physical power—and oh, the power you'll discover there!

If your physical self constitutes only one one-thousandth of you, do you want to live in and of that tiny fraction of yourself? Or do you choose to let *all* of you, your Expanded Self, live your life right here on Earth? Easy question.

All the limitless resources of your Infinite Self are available to you in every moment. The only question is, are you tuned to it vibrationally or is the physical world grabbing too much of your attention and distracting you from what's most real? Are you allowing, aware, and appreciative of your Larger Resources?

Just as in my previous book, there is no work to do; there is only evolution and expansion—joyful, constant, and ongoing. And the more you focus on your Non-Physical Self, the more of You becomes accessible to You. Your Large Self doesn't need to be worked on—just step into it more.

Summarizing: to build your power of intention, appreciate yourself as the vast Non-Physical being you are rather than limiting yourself to your visible physical being and your physical capacities only.

Get all of you to the party.

ACTIVITY: Meditation - Appreciate your Non-Physical Self.
There is an audio of this in Level Two.

- Close your eyes, smile lightly, and breathe softly.
- Place all of your conscious attention on your breathing.
- Deliberately appreciate the simple, blissful sensation of breathing.
- Imagine your breath as a mystical bridge between the physical and the Non-Physical.
- Appreciate the mystery of breathing, how it occurs without any thought or effort throughout your entire life.
- Now, allow yourself to drop deep down into the core of your being, to the place where your breath is sustained by a mere intention of your Non-Physical Large Self.
- Go deeper, beyond space and time; go where you originated as an intention—when an intention was shot into the Fertile Void, seeding the Creation of You.
- Breathe, and feel your Large, Infinite Self surrounding you.
- Appreciate the vast, Larger part of You that is Non-Physical.
- Stay in this state as long as you like, then come back to the physical refreshed.

Identify with your Non-Physical Self,
that vastly Larger, more all-knowing aspect of you.

* * * * * * * *

What Focus Is

As a professor aims a laser pointer at the chalkboard to draw her students' attention to the point she's making, the pointer helps them focus more sharply.

Think of your mind as a laser pointer you use to focus your power. When you aim your mind at something, your consciousness follows it, and your power flows there.

While The Presence has the incomprehensibly unlimited power to be everywhere at once, we humans are focusing machines. The human mind can't hold awareness of the entire Universe all at once. Researchers say most humans can't hold more than seven thoughts in mind at one time. Even when we say we're multi-tasking, what we're really doing is jumping from one focus to another.

People who have cosmic awareness experiences of being one with everything and experiencing everything at once cannot sustain that for very long at this stage of human evolution. While they are in those states, most people have difficulty functioning in the ordinary world.

As a physical human, you focus from your own perspective, in your own singular way, creating an experience that is unique in all the Universes. You point your consciousness at things, and that attention either aligns your vibration with what you're looking at, or you more powerfully bring that situation into alignment with what you want.

Be The Most Powerful Component

Before gaining mastery, you are more reactive than proactive or creative. Other people and circumstances determine your feelings. Genetics and the environment determine your health, and you need medicine to fix things that go awry with your body.

Other vibrations can overwhelm you when you are not the most powerful component in your reality. You particularly need to watch where you point that thing, because you can't yet hold your own vibration without getting knocked off center. You tend to align with the world outside by default.

With mastery, the world outside aligns with you. You are the most powerful component. No matter what other people or circumstances offer you, you keep returning to your own center. You determine your own vibration.

Like Jesus, today's powerful healers and teachers don't "buy" a person's illness or story—when we look at them all we see is their wholeness and perfection, so illness and issues cannot stand up to that truth. Our aligned vibration pulls the ill person's vibration into alignment, if they'll allow it.

As your power of intention expands, you become the most powerful component in most situations—you exert the strongest influence. That's why some people can look at or deal with difficult things and stay up—they're the most powerful component.

When you're helping someone who's in a lower vibration, they come up rather than you going down. If there's a conflict, you intend that your vibration invites both of you to be your Large Selves. You entice the other to come up to your level rather than letting them take you downward.

Give yourself room to be human as you play with this, and be compassionate to yourself if you let something knock you off center. Mastery isn't perfection—it's always being able to get back on center.

The most powerful component in an interaction prevails.

Power is the ability to have an effect. Power is intrinsically neither good nor bad. Power of intention allows you to vibrate your desire powerfully enough that it must materialize for you.

Being the most saintly or the most "right" component isn't the same as being the most powerful component. You can be "good" and "right" and the other person who "isn't" can prevail. Good or bad, saintly or evil, right or wrong are irrelevant parameters when it comes to the power of intention. Being good gets you nothing.

Being good, saintly, or right gets you nothing.

We are worthy and good right now, even in our human imperfection. If you don't yet feel that in your bones, intend to claim your worthiness now. When you truly feel your worthiness and goodness, you allow yourself to claim your power of intention. If you think you're not worthy, Life must agree with you, and thus you hold yourself back. Unworthiness is a literal mis-take.

Two definitions of integrity offered by the Random House dictionary are useful in understanding how to claim your power of intention:

in·teg·ri·ty

1. the state of being whole, entire, or undiminished: "to preserve the integrity of the empire."

You want to be whole, all of one mind, and not contradicted or divided within yourself. You are at one with your desire or intention.

2. a sound, unimpaired, or perfect condition: "the integrity of a ship's hull."

You want to be strong, unbreakable, and impenetrable when faced with obstacles or outside forces.

Pulse complete integrity with your desire.

When I lead the Five-Day Silent Retreat, for example, I vibrate in complete integrity with my desire for the participants claim their power and depart transformed. People arrive in various states, and, while I observe and feel that in a general way, I don't focus on their problems *at all.* I don't even know their problems, and I certainly don't process them through their problems—that would focus us on what's "wrong." I see them as who they really are: whole and strong. My Large Self sees only their greatest potential and the shortest route to it.

I hold an undivided, un-contradicted, high frequency vortex that strongly magnetizes them to join me. I am the most powerful component; therefore my intention prevails despite their doubts and fears. As they let go and approach this vortex, it sweeps them in, and magic begins to happen.

This is not "power *over*," but "power to." It's pure power that radiates, invites, magnetizes, and influences without force or attachment. Intend to be the most powerful component in your world.

On the fifth day, the final initiation awakens participants' power to heal and give powerful Divine Openings. When people ask me how that initiation works, perhaps they're expecting to hear that I use some esoteric process or magical metaphysical keys. I tell them, "It happens purely by intention." I am clear and devoid of doubt, so it has never failed, even with people who thought they surely wouldn't get it. Their free will choices do determine how quickly or slowly they progress after we part.

My Large Self does the work, not my limited human self. I don't have the compulsion to define it or understand it with my mind. My greatest gift may be my ability to keep my limiting mind *out* of my work.

Undivided, undiminished integrity and clarity are huge components of the power of intention. My certainty comes not from faith, but from many years of letting go to The Presence and seeing the *evidence.*

This book exists in a vibrational vortex that gently but surely invites you to let go and vibrate at that frequency. When you do, it feels good, and your power of intention increases. No amount of work helps—but relaxing releases resistance and allows energy to flow more freely.

Yes, I'm inviting you to do nothing, and know nothing. How easy is that?

Intellectual understanding is a consolation prize
you could settle for instead of miracles.

Stop. Lightly ponder what you've read, then let go and let your mind take a relaxing vacation.

* * * * * * * *

What Materialism Really Is

At age nine, Goldie Hawn made a decision to always be happy. People would say, "What do you want to be when you grow up?" She'd answer, "I want to be happy."

Pressing on, they'd inquire, "Do you want to be a dancer, an actress?" She'd maintain, "I want to be happy." Goldie was one of those rare people who knew at an early age that *how you feel* is the primary thing—that if you are happy, life is good.

Feelings are the treasure we possessed all along, but we undervalued or ignored them, thinking other people, places, and things held the keys to our fulfillment. That is *materialism.*

Materialism is thinking, feeling, and living as if you're nothing but a physical body. The flesh and bone material aspect of you is a tiny fraction of who you are, although it's cherished in the Non-Physical. Value your human body and the physical world; just identify yourself *more* with the larger Non-Physical reality.

Having nice things isn't necessarily materialistic. There is absolutely no judgment from The Presence about having wildly extravagant material things. People might make you wrong, especially spiritual people who talk about wanting abundance but have subtle judgments of it!

Materialism goes at manifestation backwards, focusing on the material people, places, experiences, and things we think we *must have* to get the feeling—and since it gives too much power to the material world—*that's* materialism.

Everyone knows relationships, jobs, cars, travel, health, friends, and homes are wonderful manifestations, but feelings are much easier and faster to create. Feelings are the one thing you're totally in control of each and every moment! Yes, feelings are pre-manifestational indicators, but they are also manifestational end products.

Feelings are actual manifestations, desirable ends in themselves.

Take the non-materialistic route just because it works better and feels better, and the speeded up materialization is just a bonus. If you focus first on how you feel, those Instrument Panel readings guide you to what you truly desire. Your true heart's desire may be different than your limited mind could conceive of.

Here's the first revelation toward building your power of intention: *feelings are manifestations in and of themselves.* Feeling good is actually the most valuable jackpot manifestation imaginable, yet people can discount it or fail to appreciate it. Feeling good is an achievement in and of itself.

With the help of Divine Openings you can change your feelings pretty fast. A material change may take a while longer, or it might come quickly, but you can be happy in the meantime.

When people say to me in a counseling series, "Well, I feel great, but nothing's happened. I'm still in debt," I say, "Feeling good is what you thought getting out of debt would get you. That's the real reason you wanted out of debt—to feel good—and now *you feel great*! Hello! Appreciate this with all your heart!"

People talk about their ship coming in? Once you're feeling better, your ship *is on its way in*, and not appreciating that makes it turn right around and go back out to sea. Don't miss the boat, darlin'.

When you not only don't appreciate but also actively reject your accomplishment by making the good feeling not enough, you delay or completely reverse the materialization you say you desire. Value the feelings most of all.

No one would ever yell at the fireplace, "Give me heat if you want me to give you any wood!" That's crazy. Yet people will demand the outer world and other people must change before they can feel better. That's just as crazy. Anyone can feel good when the world is doing what they want, but when you can feel good no matter what the outer world is temporarily doing, that's mastery. You're on your way to a great life.

You want fire? Give it the fuel it needs.

Anne wanted a great new relationship, because she wanted to be happier, and couldn't be happy until the relationship arrived. Another woman, Betty, was ready for a great relationship too, but she'd been doing Divine Openings for about a year, so she decided to get happy about relationship first. Both wanted the feeling of happiness.

Betty went straight for happiness and *got it now*. She was aware that she needed to raise her vibration about past relationships, but she didn't work on herself, she just intended it. She began enjoying her life, and started taking new job training and having more fun. She joked that she was going to get started dating at some point in her busy life, and would probably have to kiss a few toads; but that was never necessary. One day recently a man from her apartment complex knocked on her door and asked her out! They've been together ever since, and it's easy and compatible.

Anne, by going at it materially, made her happy feeling dependent on some future time when she materializes a man—but it's hard to attract a happy man from a lack-ful, unfulfilled vibrational state.

My definition of materialism isn't judgmental, nor does it make this wondrous material world wrong or inferior. I use the word materialism to distinguish whether we're focusing on the eternal Non-Physical and the feelings that guide us from Large Self, or on the mere physical.

Source never judges you.

At the heart of spiritual anti-materialism is a well-intentioned effort to get people to value the Source of all things rather than worship the things themselves. It went too far to the other extreme, and made the physical and material world *wrong* or *evil* or something to *ascend out of*. We created this realm deliberately for the physical experience, and to express in physical embodiment, so how could the material world possibly be wrong?

Physical is great and to build your maximum power of intention, focus on what is real, enduring, and profound: your Non-Physical, eternal Self.

Don't worship the gift.
Worship the Giver.

Hundreds of people have written me that before Divine Openings there were so many things that had to happen before they could get happy: make more money, get a better house, find their true love, settle a lawsuit, or their family had to act a different way.

Then by just going along and doing Divine Openings they got happy without all those things, and they're still happy whether those things have shown up or not.

This is huge. Feeling better is not just step one in the materialization process—it's everything. Make more space for this deep in your consciousness, right now, because when you truly focus on the

Non-Physical, you get to be happy right now, *and* you release resistance and build your power of intention. It's the mega-bonus jackpot people think winning the lottery would bring.

Manifesting a better feeling tips the entire Universe.

Being a powerful Conscious Creator has brought me many nice things: a beautiful home, a paid off truck and horse trailer, horses and money to feed them even when hay has become outrageously expensive, lovely clothes, some vacations, and the money to finance all of my own work without investors. I haven't carried any debt except for a home mortgage in years, and my taxes and monthly bills are always happily and appreciatively paid *early*. As I pay them I deeply, viscerally appreciate the services and products that money bought.

I'm not itching to make millions—that's just not me. There's no resistance to money, or judgment of money. However much money anyone wants is fine. It's just clear more money wouldn't bring me more happiness. I already have happiness and it continues to spiral gently upward. I'm in control of it, it's not an accident, and no one can take it away.

Studies show that wealth beyond covering basic needs *does not increase happiness*. I'm not one of those authors who promise you'll make a million dollars next year, although you very well could if it's right for you. If you use what this book says I do promise you that you'll be happier and more powerful in a year, and it will continue to expand steadily.

While horseback riding I heard strain in the voice of my friend as she expressed a desperate desire to pay off her debt. I tossed out, "Get happy *with* your debt." It was an entirely new concept that she could be just as happy today as the day she pays it off.

Debt is just a story. To help people reframe how they *feel* about debt I'll quip, "Wow, people just *gave you that money*—on your word, for nothing! They didn't take your firstborn child or anything! And they can't lock you up or kill you if you don't pay it! How freaking fantastic is that?"

Huge corporations and countries are in unbelievable debt. It's just a funny money game to those guys—I promise you money isn't all that real to them. Donald Trump's debt payments probably equal the budget of a third world country. This perspective flips a scary story to appreciation, even humor.

Money Ease, a wonderful audio in the Self-Paced Level Two Online Retreat correlates well with this section. It also applies to gaining ease in any area of life.

Create A New Matrix

This section is short, but it's a core piece of power of intention, and we'll play with it again and again throughout the book. Whenever you think, feel, and pulse a signal, you create a Non-Physical template, or matrix of your intention or desire, or its opposite.

You might picture the matrix looking somewhat like graph paper, except it's not two-dimensional, it's multi-dimensional, and it's invisible.

Imagine that its little lines act like magnets that magnetize the perfect physical elements and components to fill the little empty cubes in the matrix.

With your thoughts, feelings, and the pulse you're broadcasting, you create the *general* lines of the Non-Physical matrix, and then leave it to The Presence to make sure the *specific* physical details are magnetized to it. The end products—the materializations, events, and people that show up always conform to the matrix you created.

> *Thoughts and feelings form the matrix your*
> *creation or materialization is built upon.*

When you focus on what you want to feel and experience, information, resources, and circumstances are magnetized to that matrix. Feeling and thinking about what you don't want, stressing, worrying, and pulsing lower vibrations creates a matrix too, and it fills in with physical elements that match those vibrations.

> *Go straight to The Source of all materializations,*
> *the Non-Physical.*

* * * * * * * *

Attention Creates

Gangsters as well as spiritual masters can master the power of intention, so once again, how spiritual or good you are has nothing to do with what we're talking about here. You might as well drop the judgments and limitations of stereotypical spirituality—it won't help you build your power of intention.

Do I have a lot of what is usually called "spiritual power?" Yes, but it may not be what you think it is. It is Non-Physical, vibratory power that transcends the physical world even as we live in the physical world. The more powerful you get, the more quickly things manifest, and the more conscious you must be of where you point that thing.

Focusing on a problem is completely different from focusing on solutions and possibilities. When you point your attention at the problem long enough, it inadvertently forms a matrix. Your attention has laser-strength power. "How would that mess happen?" you might wonder, "I was merely concerned about this problem!" Your attention fuels it with your power and juice.

> *Your attention becomes a matrix.*
> *Watch where you point that thing!*

You may think you're focusing on something in order to solve it, but check to be sure. If it lowers your vibration, it is influencing you more than you're influencing it. *It's* the most powerful component.

For example, when leading the Five Day Silent Retreat, if I was not the most powerful component, a roomful of people in lower vibrational states would not transform the way they do. They might bring me down instead of me bringing them up. In your own life, when you're the most powerful component, you elevate the situation at work or in a family crisis.

We get unlimited do-overs, so don't worry about failing as you go through experiences to master this. Fly or flop, it's great feedback, and you'll adjust. Just stick to your intention to become the most powerful component, and you will get there increasingly often.

Check your Instrument Panel and feel where you are in the moment—there are no hard and fast rules here—go by *what happens and what you feel* when you interact with the world and circumstances. Relax and enjoy the unfolding of your mastery.

Be the most powerful component.

The proof of what you're vibrating is always in the results. Results are reality, at least temporarily. Fortunately, reality is fleeting and changeable—very good news for us fallible humans.

Summary: If you focus on something and *you* shift *its* vibration then you're the most powerful component in the interaction—your integrity and power of intention is strong. If a low vibration person or situation rises up to meet you where you are, you are the most powerful component. Your desire is undivided and uncompromised.

Read the above again if you're not absolutely clear on what it means to be the most powerful component. You don't have to master this today, just intend to, then rest and assimilate.

* * * * * * * *

Skip To The Payoff!

Once you embrace skipping to the payoff you're going to find it's the most powerful thing you've ever done.

When anyone asks me to help them manifest something, I tell them physical manifestations are way down the chain from where we'll be starting—they are mere by-products—and we're going to focus on something far more important. We start with manifesting the *feelings* they want. That's skipping to the payoff, and it teaches you how to do *instant manifestation*.

Focus on creating the thoughts, feelings, and the general tone of what you want rather than the specific materializations you want. Focusing on the specific material outcome too much at the start can narrow your options, where generalizing your focus opens you up to allow for limitless options. Your job is to feel good, let go of limits, and stay out of the way.

When you focus on your feelings first, you get to *skip to the payoff* and feel good *now*. The physical materialization might take a little while—but in the meantime you're feeling good and enjoying life. When you manifest the feeling you imagined that material thing, person, or circumstance would give you, you get… what … you … wanted … right … now.

It's instant manifestation!

You can create feelings pretty quickly and enjoy them now. You get instant manifestation, which gives you more confidence, which builds over time: if I can do that I can do even more! That releases more resistance, and then good things cascade. Wow!

Skip to the payoff you really wanted: to feel good.

Here's what you don't want to do—a vicious cycle:

- You create a good feeling, then check to see if your physical manifestation has come yet, and if it hasn't, you lose the good feeling and you're back at square one.
- So you create the good feeling again, then check to see if your manifestation has come yet, and if it hasn't, you lose the good feeling and you're back at square one.
- So you create the good feeling again, then check to see if your manifestation has come yet, and if it hasn't, you lose the good feeling and you're back at square one.

A new desire is always exciting, expansive, and energizing. But too often, if it doesn't show up fast enough vibration drops. Your job is to find every way you can to think, feel, and authentically pulse that reality *now*.

There is no surer way to delay materialization than stressing or straining about it—that's called *getting in the way*. If you manage to get the things you wanted without raising your vibration, having them may not even give you the good feeling you though it would.

Savor the waiting and keep yourself soothed. Make it your intention above all to feel good—or at least feel a little better about it—right now.

Here's a *virtuous* (not a vicious) cycle—you stay focused on feeling good rather than taking score.

- The better you feel the better things get.
- The better things get the better you feel.
- The better you feel the better things get.
- The better things get the better you feel.
- And the better you feel the better things get.
- And the better things get the better you feel. Need I go on?

Because I'm adept at materializing things quickly I particularly must pay attention to how I feel.

Since to feel good is what we actually want when we intend any materialization, the feeling is the primary manifestation to focus upon. It becomes more important than the material outcome we thought we had to have. Feeling better is not just a step in the materialization process, it's the whole point—it's the payoff I was looking for in the first place.

The feeling itself is a powerful manifestation to celebrate!

If the old reality is emotionally gripping, it can be harder to drop the old story and feel the better feelings needed to create the new matrix. I found making up a story starring someone else with a similar desire flipped the switch for me—I suddenly possessed the objectivity to imagine the new scenario. I was careful not to get attached to the details—the point was to generate powerfully compelling good feelings to create the new matrix and the new reality.

Just write your own new scene. Here's an example: Paul was in a bind. His mortgage was due, and he'd just lost his job. He felt hopeless to find the money, but he knew to drop that story and feel the feeling—he felt just a bit better and went to visit his sister. A friend of his sister's dropped by; she was in town looking for a place to live in that area for six months while her husband worked on an assignment. Paul offered to rent them his house and he would find a place to stay for that period. His sister offered that he could use her guestroom and do some repairs she desperately needed done. The rent not only covered his mortgage, but his food and gas costs. Everyone was served. Paul got a great job within two months, stashed away some savings, and moved back into his home after six months. His savings grew steadily for the first time in his life.

It's easier for you to buy into that reality because it's not about you—it's just a story so the mind doesn't negate it! Notice it feels real enough to generate feelings in you, and that's the power of it. The better feelings move you out of your impossible situation and into the realm of possibility. I laughed when I realized my fictional story always made me smile instantly, where if I tried to imagine me in that new story I got sucked back into the old reality that was so emotionally intense.

* * * * * * * *

What Is Reality?

Now let's really dive in. Until you deliberately commit to focus on the subtle Non-Physical, your senses are tuned to pick up only the gross physical inputs of sight, sound, smell, hearing, and physical sensations, and those are extremely distracting. Regularly take your focus off the physical for a while and intend to feel the more subtle Non-Physical vibrations. You can do it—this book will guide you.

What's most real and enduring is not what grabs most of our attention. What is most real is the Larger, Non-Physical aspect of reality that sources, fuels, causes, creates, and encompasses the physical reality—it's invisible and it does not usually demand our focus—we each must choose it consciously, daily. Otherwise we get the default reality that is completely physically focused, visible, tangible, visceral, right in our face, hard to ignore, that too often distracting us from our Non-Physical knowing and power.

The physical world often distracts us from
that which is most real and powerful.

There's no denying it's challenging to keep your focus on the true power of your Non-Physical Self when your very physical self is hurting, your very physical lover has just left, or your very physical bills need to be paid. It's all too tempting to give all our attention to physical world on a daily basis, and all our *power* too. The physical world is designed to be grippingly real.

Sometimes the most precious treasure is hidden in the last place we'd ever think to look. People often seek answers and grasp for salvation outside themselves for decades while The Non-Physical Presence that creates everything is quietly pulsing within them, and in everything, everywhere around them.

Beginners or even spiritually advanced people just beginning Divine Openings ask me about how to apply it to living in the Real World. My first response is always to laugh! *There is no Real World!* There is only the one you create.

There is *no single objective reality.* What you're currently experiencing as reality is what you created with your past thoughts, feelings, and the collective reality you bought into before you knew better. That's all it is. While it is solid and real for all practical purposes, it's temporary. Don't give it too much weight. It can change very fast once you create a new matrix.

Your world is your creation—always was, always will be.

Here's an example of a time I just would not buy the reality I was seeing, and so it changed. On the way to drop my mom off at LAX airport, it appeared we'd left her wallet somewhere—not good news if you need your ID to board a plane. I'll usually refuse to buy too quickly into a reality like that—I virtually expect it to shift instantly for me, but at the same time, I keep the intention light as the touch of a gnat's wing, and try not to resist whatever may occur.

"I never lose anything! You couldn't lose your wallet when you're with me!" I insisted confidently. Before flying into fearful actions like speeding back to the last place she had her wallet out, I sat and breathed to get in my power and find a centered, calm feeling.

I had just looked all over the car in every nook and cranny a minute ago and it wasn't there, but the next time I looked, her wallet appeared between the car seats. When I stay calm, that's just how it usually goes. When it doesn't go that way, I look for how it's right the way it did go.

You don't have to live in the collective consciousness's version of the Real World—there are literally unlimited versions of Real Worlds you can play in, and we won't even debate whether they're real or illusory. They feel real when you're living them!

Intend to:

- Focus on the Non-Physical more than the physical.
- Stubbornly identify yourself as your powerful Large Self, not your limited human self.
- Feel good first.
- Know what you see today is only what you created yesterday—it can change in the wink of an eye when you create a new matrix.
- Relax and let go to the flow.

Even after Grace has lifted you, what happens after that depends *entirely* on you since have Free Will. You can stay in Grace, go jump in a slime pit, stick one foot in Grace and the other in a slime pit, or anything in between.

You can wrangle with the Real World, or by intending how you want to feel create another matrix that feels better to you. Your Large Self is always pulsing the solution, the peace, the love, and the bliss you want. There's nothing to do to get there—just intend.

If we make the physical world and what happens in it more real to us than the Non-Physical, and make the physical world our God, power is forfeited. You are "made in His image" as a Creator. As you step into creating purely by intention, you claim your heritage. You're either a Conscious Creator, or a Sponge that soaks up whatever happens to be there. You can't be both.

I don't respect reality all that much—it's all temporary—especially if I don't like it.

Watch where you point that thing.

ACTIVITY: Greet The Day

Each day when you awake, greet the physical day *and* the Non-Physical Source of it with a little smile as you snuggle yourself in your bed. As you appreciate the sun, rain, or fog, acknowledge the Non-Physical Source that created it, of which you are a part.

Have a chat with The Presence about the upcoming day. Create your relationship with the Non-Physical Creator to be casual, friendly, and personal—not nebulous, because when it's personal, your power of intention is more potent. You were shown how to create an intimate, personal concept of God, your Non-Physical Self, while reading *Things Are Going Great In My Absence*. If it is not yet real to you, review that now before you proceed.

Intend alignment with your Large Self each morning. It doesn't matter if you do the day perfectly or not. You get unlimited do-overs.

* * * * * * * *

It's About Who You're Being

You think it, desire it, or dream it, and to the extent you're accessing the unlimited power of your Non-Physical Large Self on that subject, it appears. It's easy and automatic to dream, to ask, to want. If you're in the habit of being your Large Self, operating on that cosmic cruise control, having it appear is also easy. If you're out of alignment with your Large Self on a topic, no amount of action can make up for that.

Your greatest power is in your Non-Physical Large Self, which brings us back to one of our main themes: identify yourself more *as* your Large Self. In the Non-Physical we "be" and create, but don't "do." We created ourselves in the physical to "do," take actions, and have physical adventures—but as the clever saying goes, when you're good with a hammer, everything looks like a nail—so humans tend to leap to action first. We do first and intend second or not at all; act first and consider how we're vibrating second; speak first, think second.

Turn all that around.

Consider who you're being before doing anything. I don't mean are you being all spiritual—I mean are you expanded and powerful, open-hearted and clear? Shift gears if needed, expand into Large Self, and use pure intention and just a little patience before contemplating massive action.

Who do you think you are? Teachers and parents may have used that question to shame and humble you when you were a child. I'm using it to expand you, to invite you to step up and be the Large being you actually are. If you feel too small or humble, there is so much more of you to live into.

Sure, we're human and fallible, but fortunately we don't have to be completely expanded or perfect to have enormous power of intention. It's enough to be strongly committed to stay awake and be. Intend now to "be" your Large Self more of the time, and furthermore to *identify yourself as* your Large Self.

Intention first, action second.

Who we're being and vibrating is more important than what we're doing and saying. When we're being our more limited selves, we have only our finite human capacities and resources to rely on. When we're being our Large Selves we have more of our infinite Non-Physical resources available, and our intentions materialize more quickly and reliably.

A teacher in another program once told me she wanted a mate that she didn't have to be enlightened with all the time. She wanted the luxury of being able to let down and be sloppy, as if it's hard "work" to stay awake! Of course the program she taught did make getting enlightened and living the good life a lot of hard work, so I can see why she felt that.

In my experience being my small self is hard work—it's not relaxing at all—it's Hell. Resisting the flow of Life is hard work. Being awake and in the flow is pure pleasure and ease. If you catch yourself dragging that old working on yourself paradigm into this, or making evolution hard—stop—that has no place here, and it holds you back. Let this be a fun game.

This is about living as your Larger or more Expanded Self as much of the time as you can, while not expecting to be perfect, and embracing your humanity and others'.

The very nature of Life is to try to shower us with abundant good, which points up the other of the two mains themes of this book: staying out of the way so things can go great in your absence. As we progress through the delightful journey of this book, you'll experience all the pieces falling into place—you'll identify yourself more and more as your Large Self, and you'll get more and more out of the way.

Take a deep, delicious breath and know there is nothing to "do" except relax, experience, and enjoy.

* * * * * * * *

What Is Being Your Large Self?

What is being your Large Self or Expanded Self? It certainly isn't trying to be "good" or perfect—that will get you off track and you can end up being a "good" victim, or actually end up out of alignment with your Large Self by using outer societal or human standards instead of aligning with what you feel is best.

Being "good" is subjective and human-judgment-based, and it doesn't build your power of intention. It's too outer-focused. When you're living as your Large Self and are inner focused and directed, you are *naturally good* and don't intentionally harm others.

Rather than checking to see if you're being good, it's more practical and useful to use your Instrument Panel to check on your alignment with your Large Self. You can clearly define whether you're in alignment or not by how you feel on your Instrument Panel (you hopefully gained facility with your Instrument Panel in *Things Are Going Great In My Absence*.)

It's more about who you're being
than what you're doing.

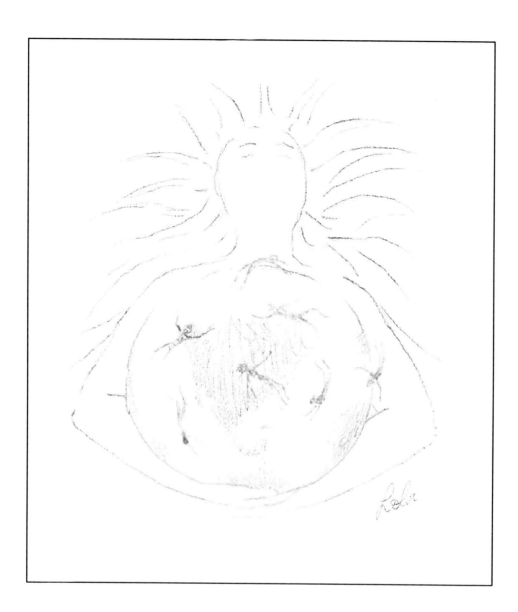

ACTIVITY: Intend To Focus On What Is Real

If you ever find you're letting current, temporary (it's always temporary) physical reality distract you and usurp your power, play this game to access your full power and build your power of intention:

- Intend yourself into Large Self Perspective.
- Expand your awareness of You as Larger and more eternal than any fleeting physical manifestation that has your attention.
- As you intend focus on that Large perspective, it grows effortlessly.
- Intend to "temporarily stop the words in your head." Try it. It works.
- Observe any temporary physical reality as your Large Self experiences it, noticing how the physical situation is now much, much smaller than You. As you practice this you form a new habit.

Once you're in your power what you want begins to line up in the pre-manifest, Non-Physical realm where every creation, wanted or unwanted, originates. In other words, create the template in the Non-Physical, and the physical form must build on it (it is Law).

The hard way is to try to change things solely at the level of physical work and action. Even trying to think it into being is too much work. Line up with your Large Self's unlimited, all-powerful perspective and let the physical materialization line up with that—much easier than pushing rocks up hills.

Hardest of all is to try to force the physical manifestation to go against any resistant vibration you might have going right now. That's like you pushing the rock from one side while your resistance pushing it from the other side.

Something has to give. Let it be you. In Large Self perspective you have no resistance to your own desires.

* * * * * * * *

The Real Meaning Of "You Reap What You Sow"

In *Things Are Going Great In My Absence,* I talk about how once-puzzling passages from scriptures I read in childhood suddenly made sense to me after my awakening. Now the passage, "You reap what you sow," is clear to me. It doesn't mean if you are bad you get punished, or if you're good you get rewarded. You can look around and see that's not true!

What it does mean is that how you're vibrating (the seed) determines what things and experiences are attracted into your reality (what you sow.) It has nothing to do with being good or bad. A person being selfless and generous but vibrating victim energy will get hurt, robbed, or taken advantage of. A criminal vibrating positively about having money and pleasure will have it. A criminal vibrating guilt will get arrested. A psychopath who has no guilt may never be caught, but you don't have to worry about him unless you're vibrating victimhood, unworthiness, or guilt.

I often say things several different ways because feedback from people tells me some people hear it best one way and others hear it best another way.

There are many ways the vibrational seeds of lack of money might have been planted in you: by parental or societal conditioning, by complaining about lack of money, continuing to vibrate victim after losing a job or getting robbed, vibrating fear about money, giving it power, making it evil, judging rich people, and so on. Many spiritual paths make money wrong, so it's no wonder so many spiritual people are money-repellent (sometimes I call it allergic to money.) Your Large Self allows you to vibrate however you want, without judgment.

Someone deep in money lack might contract into small-self perspective when the very thought of money comes up. No matter how the money lack got started, rather than try to fix your small self, just shift into your Large Self perspective, and you vibrate differently. Your Large Self has no issues, fears, or limitations.

Again, this works when you've first prepared and mastered the basics in *Things Are Going Great In My Absence*. If you haven't, this will be frustrating and you'll complain it didn't work. We told up front!

Using another analogy, an architectural one, the intention is the architect's initial thought and inspiration to build a building. The intention is the Non-Physical blueprint that guides the construction of the physical building. Then his blueprint is filled in with the essential people, resources, and building materials he needs to make a physical building.

You don't expect to get a mansion if you give your builder the blueprint for a barn. Similarly you can't expect to get a prosperous life if you hand The Presence a blueprint for poverty, for example: fear, struggle, heaviness, unworthiness and lack.

You can't overcome your own vibration no matter how hard you try to push that rock up that hill. Turn those daunting things over to The Presence if they're too big for you.

Your intention is right now drawing up a blueprint, creating a matrix, for tomorrow's creation, and physical things and experiences will be assembled to fit that.

Your intention, conscious or not, forms a matrix.
Materialization fleshes it out.

Remember that intention creates instantly. Everyone already can and does already do it. They just don't always know *how they're doing it*. You grow your power of intention as you get clearer about what you're vibrating, and better at reading your Instrument Panel.

I recently gave a phone session to a sophisticated, cultured man who was at the time in prison for life, convicted of a crime he said he didn't commit. He had read the book *The Secret*, and had created everything he ever wanted and more, and then his whole life fell apart. Prior to our session, he'd been puzzled as to why and how he had created his devastating downfall, although he was perfectly willing to claim that he created it.

As I guided him through a process from the Jumping The Matrix Self-Paced Online Retreat, his Large Self quickly took him to the crucial moment when his perfect life started spiraling downward. He saw himself in his formerly perfect life with his perfect family, and experienced the very moment when he suddenly felt he was unworthy of it all, and began to systematically unravel it as he lost his job, family, dream home, marriage, and then became involved with a dysfunctional woman, culminating in serious charges and imprisonment.

Just imagine, with all that manifestational power and knowledge, worthiness was his blind spot—the counter-intention that undid it all. Although he'd learned the materialization process quite well, he had no relationship with his Larger Non-Physical Self—he was entirely materially focused. When a path neglects the bigger part of who you are, it's hollow and insubstantial.

I guided him to an alternate reality where another version of him felt worthy and so remained in that former, happy life. The session helped him literally change his reality over the next five months, resulting in the conviction being overturned—he was released without mounting any appeals (which he couldn't afford to do), something attorneys assured him never happens—a true miracle.

When you shift, your past, present, and future also shift.

Go to DivineOpenings.com/testimonials if you'd like to read the story in his own words, with his identity concealed.

* * * * * * * *

Claim More Of Your Non-Physical Power

In the game of hide and seek we come here eager to play, the knowledge that we are God focused into many physical forms is made taboo. Of course, we like the game and don't want it to be over too soon, but we're also drawn to the relief of awakening.

There's more to it than just awakening and remembering who we are. Each time in each new life that we go to sleep and awaken again, it's not just a monotonous circling around then "coming home again." There's a forward progression and expansion that fuels evolution—that's driven both by the tension and contrast created by forgetting and longing to remember, and the pull of the joy of expanding into our next full potential.

Each time we play this game of slumbering to awaken again, the Universe is expanded by the desires that blast out from us in our passion to have things be ever better.

God-Realization is a term some traditions use for living as a human who is fully aware of being God, and who has access to that power in this life, but like all other concepts, it can be confusing because there are so many contradictory definitions out there.

The dragons that guard the cave entrance where the treasure is hidden are: unworthiness, feeling small, self-limitation, fear, and thoughts like, "Oh, I can't possibly be that Large and wise and wonderful." A client recently went to church with her parents in Ireland and was shocked at how many of the ancient prayers had the congregation intoning how unworthy they were. She didn't chant along!

There's a natural progression that expands from you having a *relationship with* The Presence, which implies separation, to knowing yourself *as* The Presence. So many who have been doing Divine Openings for a while tell me it now feels as if they're talking to themselves rather than some exalted being. They've come to know themselves as The Presence in a human body not just in theory, but also in experience.

Whenever we pray, begging God for something, we're sending out a broadcast that says, "I am separate from God, and powerless to create," or worse, "I am a victim." We create a separation that isn't there. Speak your intention, knowing it is done.

At this place in your evolution your power of intention increases dramatically. You're no longer "asking God" for manifestations or mercy, like a child asking for permission or a prisoner begging for release—you're a budding Conscious Creator exercising your ever-increasing creative power. "Letting go to The Presence" just means letting go to the Larger part of You that's unlimited and has no resistance, not to some "other" or authority figure you must please.

You begin to operate consciously on a continuum of being more or less in alignment with your Largest Self in any given moment. You're either more or less expanded. You don't make it wrong to be contracted or out of alignment, because you know that the very tension and contrast of being out of alignment provides powerful stimulation to expand yourself and the Universe even more.

If I had to identify one factor that most increases your power of intention it would be that you experience yourself as The Creator expressing in your physical body. Creators create! You grow your power by primarily intending that feeling and that state of being, and life gets better and better. It's only a side effect that you get better at letting material manifestations show up, and savoring the waiting till they do.

Just keep moving and stay awake.

* * * * * * * *

Enlightenment vs. Seeking

Once your enlightenment begins unfolding you will expand constantly and eternally as long as you allow it to happen and don't get in the way *too* much. Simply intend to stay awake, be willing to feel, and take it within, and you'll evolve as fast as you can handle it. Many people even ask to have it slow down!

I said at the beginning of the book that building your power of intention is more about what you *don't do* than what you do. Here is a major component of mastering the power of intention: *you can't get to a high level of mastery while still seeking and processing.*

Resist if you must. Rationalize it any way you want to. Do what you choose. This is not a judgment, nor an edict—I just tell you what I see working, and not working, for thousands of people. That's what I do every day.

If I'm preaching to the choir here—if you've ceased seeking or never were a spiritual or personal development modality junkie, congratulations! You're going to go higher *because of what you're not doing.* Read this part just to enjoy and celebrate where you are, and to laugh; it is funny.

I said some of this in *Things Are Going Great In My Absence,* so why am I saying it again? Like other things I said in that book, people don't hear what they're not ready to hear, sometimes even after reading it several times. There will be some of you who've been pushing rocks up hills, are tired, and are finally ready to hear this now.

In a recent session a very smart, entrepreneurial businesswoman said she read the book three times before she could begin to hear what I was saying about the Instrument Panel and some other things. Parts of it were so foreign to her reality, the book might as well have been written in Farsi. It wasn't penetrating through the old dense reality yet. "I just didn't get it... until I started listening to the audios in Level One Online," she admitted.

Listening with old paradigm ears, trying to make it fit into the old paradigm was never going to work. She stuck with it, and was glad she did. She recognized and let go of old paradigm concepts, beliefs, and clichés, and it all began to work for her. I acknowledged and appreciated her willingness to stick with it, and give herself time to let it in.

People I meet often ask, "Well, what can I compare Divine Openings to?" This is equal to "What box can I toss it into so I don't have to experience anything new?" I reply, "It's not like anything else you know." Blank expressions greet me as their minds struggle with that, as if to say, "It *has* to be like something I already *know!*"

If someone tries Divine Openings, but lets his mind cram it into an existing box with all the other stuff he's collected in his metaphysical kitchen junk drawer, it distorts, dilutes, and shrinks their perception of it.

Even the advanced sometimes unconsciously parrot New Age clichés and old paradigm concepts to me in their first couple of sessions. The very direct Cowgirl Guru in me brings awareness to that, and even if at first it's not what they wanted to hear, they feel the love behind it, and get the message.

When someone says, "I'm still working on it," Tom Hanks line from *A League Of Our Own* comes to mind. He said, "There's no *crying* in baseball!" but The Cowgirl Guru in me says, "There's no *working on it* in Divine Openings!"

If someone is still plodding along the old Modality of the Month path, and tells me, "Divine Openings isn't working for me," the Cowgirl Guru says, "You're not doing Divine Openings— you're doing modality soup. Of course it isn't working, and it won't ever work. When you straddle your old reality and the new one, you split your power, and your pants!"

If you listen to audios of my sessions, you know people get free only when they stop working on themselves—I've never seen anyone get free while running on the Hamster Wheel of fix, heal, clear, cleanse, and clear.

I just do what I do, see what I see, and write what I get from within, and when the emperor has no clothes on it seems obvious. I hadn't realized seeking addiction was a unique revelation until a man wrote me a long time ago and said, "Thank you for *giving a name to 'seeking addiction'*. I have seen this nowhere else. This has enlightened me." I did invent the term. No one else seems to notice, or want to notice it. I'm an expert—I used to be a serious seeking addict.

Enjoy this piece from my humor book, *Confessions Of A Cowgirl Guru:*

"The Hamster Wheel"

> I used to run on a hamster wheel constantly. It got me in really good shape, but it got frustrating and boring. It was the hamster wheel of personal and spiritual development. Looking back it seems weird that I did that for so long, but hey, we do a lot of things

for decades even though it never completely works. Like trying to change men. All your friends are doing it and no one else is getting there either, so it just seems like the thing to do and you keep doing it.

Now I'm a recovering spiritual seeker. And I don't try to change men anymore, either. I get them ready to wear, pre-washed, and pre-worn. Some other woman has done all the hard work.

Did you know I started Spiritual Seekers Anonymous seven years ago?
It's so anonymous no one knows about it.

I'd start the meetings with, "Hi, I'm Lola Jones, and I am a recovering modality junkie."

I've been clean and blissed out for almost seven years now. But one morning I woke up with the shakes and fell off the wagon. To try to steady myself, I tried counting my prayer beads while chanting the 108 sacred names of God 108 times. But it was no use—I was headed full speed toward a relapse into addictive seeking.

I called my astrologer Moon Beam Steinberg for advice, and she said, "Hey, where've you been? Mercury in retrograde is a picnic compared to what your planets are doing. STAY IN BED WITH A HELMET ON!" The helmet gave me a headache and brought up powerlessness issues, so I read three metaphysical books: on shamanism, the Kabala, and Buddhism. They were all contradictory and confused me, so I got out my crystals and cleared my chakras. I invoked the nature spirits of the trees to help me with my decision whether to go to therapeutic origami class or group therapy. All my friends would be at group therapy, so I went there and felt better hearing how f****d up they were.

There seemed to be some stagnant anger in my aura, so I floated in my salt water deprivation tank shaped like a pyramid after having a wheat grass shot to detox my liver. After that, some primal screaming blasted out my energy just enough to do some pranic healing on some past lives that came up while in the tank, giving me the inspiration to channel my dearly departed Uncle Luigi, who was an crack head dirty old man when he was incarnate, but is now one of my guides. He said, "You need to get laid, honey. Go get a love spell and a giant rose quartz crystal at your Aunt Rosaria's store, and spare no expense, you're worth it—plus her car payment is due."

I did that—not get laid, I got the love spell and the crystal—and took them to our women's empowerment group, placed them on the sacred altar, which we danced naked around while chanting and burning photos of past lovers. We painted our bodies and prayed for release of karmic attachments.

Then we had lunch.

Something still didn't feel right, I just couldn't get my bliss on, so I left a message for my massage therapist River Dolphin Rider Schwartz, but she was on a three-month walkabout with the Aborigines of Australia, studying their magic codpieces. Bummer— for me—not her. Fortunately there were some people hanging out at the Center For Anti-Apocalyptic Contemplation, and one of them gave me a serendipitous message from the Universe that I would meet my ideal lover in two years.

That was so depressing I asked my Jungian /Gestalt /Ho'oponopono /Reiki master to fit me in for a total emergency energy work-over to try to speed up my romantic progress. I came out with my hair standing on end and ran screaming (non-therapeutically) to my natural hairstylist, who communes with each follicle and only cuts the hairs that want to be cut. She shocked me by insisting I needed a perm. "Why do I need a perm?" I screeched, You don't believe in chemicals!

She shrugged, "My car payment is due."

I repeated every affirmation, mantra, and chant I knew a hundred and eight times while she worked on my hair, then went to a Spiritual Seekers Anonymous meeting to share about my relapse and recommit. It felt better to know that others too had strayed— one guy had done more modalities than I had that day. He must have gotten up earlier.

Back at home trying to meditate, I was overcome with an uncontrollable urge to sit in an essential oil bath with an ion generator to remove parasites while journaling about my childhood wounds. That got so intense I panicked and called another seeker and we practiced techniques for releasing emotional hurts until dinnertime.

Nothing was working! Finally I just drank a six-pack, smoked a joint, and ate a hamburger while watching American Idol, and all was right with the world. Thanks everybody for letting me share."

The part about smoking pot, drinking a six-pack, and eating a hamburger while watching American Idol is, of course, a joke.

I would never watch American Idol.

It's humor. I'm not serious! I'm hardly ever serious. Did I get you?

It's a good thing I'm not looking for approval or popularity, because some don't like what I teach and live in the world, but I'm invested in your freedom, not in approval. I hope you're over the need for approval too.

People would buy a lot more stuff from me if I said what they wanted to hear and didn't challenge the old paradigm, and so extended their sleepy time on the hamster wheel. But I just cannot do that. Neither can I encourage people to become dependent. I refuse to fix anything for anyone, but I set up an attractive field one can tune to that points them back home to their Large Selves, their Instrument Panel and their own power to raise their vibration. In experiencing this book, Grace assists, but you must claim your own power. I'm a catalyst. The power is already yours.

In *Things Are Going Great In My Absence* and Level One Online we offer the steps to get free of suffering and into happiness. Despite the passion I have for results, I do my best and then stay unattached to whether people let it in all the way, or not. Thankfully, the thousands of notes I get tell me Divine Openings does work—I just couldn't keep doing it if it didn't. If too many people were still not immensely better off after a couple of years, I would stop doing it.

Some continue to come visit the Divine Openings website after they get happy and free because it feels like home, they can share and celebrate, and they enjoy how it supports their ongoing expansion when so much of the world doesn't support that at all.

It's hugely rewarding to me when people tell me they've graduated to being their own teacher—that they'll always appreciate Divine Openings but don't "need" me anymore. Donna and I became good friends long distance through Divine Openings, and we talked on Skype a lot. A few years into it, after Donna had gone through Jumping The Matrix and the Five Day Retreat, Mary, another friend of hers who does Divine Openings asked her, "What Divine Openings courses are you doing now?" Donna's reply, "None. I am my own Lola now." That's the idea.

Donna sold her successful family business and is now pursuing her new passions of guiding others to fast measurable increases in their businesses, then out of the blue she started painting, and soon was selling her art. She's happy, and success is easy for her. She visits the Divine Openings website from time to time and continues to receive the newsletter because it's like news from home, and it matches her powerful new reality. She's busy living. One day I asked what was exciting her most and she wrote, "I get juice from just walking across the floor these days."

By definition, you've either realized *you're it*, or you're still *seeking it*. I say this again and again in so many ways, in the books, the audios, the videos, the sessions, until people are ready to hear it. Some people must get exhausted from beating their head against that old paradigm wall—but once they let go, Divine Openings kicks in and starts working, and life is just good.

You cannot reach a high level of mastery while still seeking.

I stopped seeking seven years ago, and my life continually rockets to new heights of love, inner peace, security, power, prosperity, and mastery without working on it. I haven't worked on myself in seven years—seriously. A few times since Divine Openings, if I tried to get rescued by someone it fortunately didn't work very well, and in that way The Presence led me back home. Being here feels really good and keeps getting better, without any more effort than staying awake.

I'm occasionally surprised to see someone achieve a high level of bliss and awareness, and then lose it by going back to seeking—literally throwing that power away. I've seen people attain high states, then follow their friends or their mind back to the old familiar herd behavior. I'll say, "There's a conscious mind piece to this. *Lead* your mind—don't *follow* it."

Your Instrument Panel gives very clear readings on the line between letting in help and giving your power away.

A master, while forever evolving, has claimed her power and is living it. A seeker is talking about it, or "learning about it," literally avoiding *the actual experience of it*. A seeker keeps the mind busily jammed with concepts, words, methods, wants, ideas, activities—any distraction rather than look and listen within. Mastery arrives when you make the space and time to go within and experience your Large Self *directly*.

This is big, so get ready: reading spiritual books, going to seminars, working on yourself, getting worked on, and doing all kinds of processes can actually *distract you from the very mastery you're seeking*.

Divine Openings always leads you back to your core, back to your own power—back inside where it always was. Divine Openings keeps reminding you to stop running around all over the world seeking and look in your own back yard, where it was all along.

* * * * * * * *

Learn To Drive

I'm sure you can relate and celebrate this with me. Many years ago, before Divine Openings, when I came up against a feeling I didn't want to feel, I'd panic and need a session. I wanted someone to fix it. Afterwards I'd feel better for a while. Then another unwanted feeling would arise and I had no clue what to do, so I needed another session. This went on almost weekly for decades.

Valuable power was being given away, but I didn't know that. Valuable feelings went unappreciated, like casting aside gold. Not knowing anything about my Instrument Panel, feelings were feared, numbed out, or ignored, and each priceless opportunity to reclaim a big chunk of power was lost.

I had strong, long-practiced vibrational habits that disempowered me in certain areas like romantic relationship. When someone "cleared" or tried to "heal" that for me, I'd just go home and vibrate the same way again—creating the same feelings, thus the same outer circumstances again. Even if it did last a while or get a little better, what power had I claimed? None.

When I didn't know I was creating it, by default I was a victim, and had no clue why things happened the way they did. Victims feel as if the power is out there—that things in life can just jump on them and hurt them. Plenty of people sympathize with the good person done wrong, and now I shudder to think how many hours were spent commiserating. We didn't know it only dug the victim hole deeper. I did learn that being the righteous victim was a huge, worthless booby prize.

Now, by claiming as light-heartedly as I can that I created it, even if I deplore what I created, I get most of my power back then and there. Without doing a thing I am suddenly a powerful Conscious Creator, not a victim. I don't have to know how I created it—that will come if it's necessary.

*Smile as you declare, "I created that
and I can create something else."*

When I first started visiting Russell in California, I was intimidated by the fast Los Angeles traffic, the maze of unfamiliar streets and freeways. After the mellow pace of Austin traffic, I felt like a granny driver in L.A.

When I'm a passenger, the routes don't stick in my mind, consequently, I didn't learn how to get anywhere by myself. I couldn't even get to the grocery store without asking Russell for directions. Nice as it was to let him drive, it was crippling my independence and ability to navigate.

Once I moved out to California, I got a navigation app on my iPhone and began to venture out on my own. Soon I had no problem driving anywhere, and one fine day suddenly found myself exhilarated while driving to the Los Angeles airport in fast, heavy traffic to pick up my mom. Then without using my navigation system at all, I intuited my way over to Hollywood to show her the sights. It was a powerful moment for me, having made that quantum leap. Remember the joy of getting your driver's license? This was that big.

I hadn't worked on it or analyzed it—it resolved naturally once I set the intention and stopped resisting.

I was free and I owned my own power.

I had learned to drive myself.

It's the same with building your power of intention. A large component of it is the ability to take the wheel of your own vibration, energy, and emotions so you have total mastery of your navigation system: the Instrument Panel.

Occasional help from others can still be wonderful, but when you navigate as your Larger Self and manage your own energy, you'll master driving. Your power of intention increases, and you can literally create yourself and your life, or recreate it as you please.

You come to read your Instrument Panel so exquisitely you can feel things coming from miles away, and can make adjustments if you don't like what you feel coming, or you can skip to the payoff— feel and enjoy the wonderful things that are coming long before they get here.

Be deliberate about this. Maybe you were hoping there was some sexy shortcut to extraordinary power of intention (shorter and easier even than Divine Openings? Seriously?)

There's a wonderful rock song I love called *Drive*, by a band oddly called Incubus. They talk about being "one of the hive," and how there's a "vague, haunting mass appeal" to being a follower and fitting in with everyone else. "It seems to be the way that everyone else gets around." He sings in a powerfully deep voice, "I'm beginning to find that I should be the one behind the wheel," then, "Hold the wheel and drive." They conclude, "But when I drive myself, my life is found. Whatever tomorrow brings, I'll be there, with open arms and open eyes."

As you hold the wheel and *drive* through your life, appreciate all of the invaluable navigational guidance your Instrument Panel gives you.

To be a powerful master of intention,
you must become your own driver.

I don't do "clearings," and I don't "heal" emotions. I don't "do" anything to people. It's wiser to teach people how to raise their vibration themselves, use Grace to lift them up, and demonstrate how to hold a higher vibration until they can do it themselves. The intention is to teach them to drive—driving them around doesn't empower them.

Someone asked, "Would you clear my house?" The answer to that question, and others like that is always, "No, your house may have lingering vibrations, but your house isn't where the power or the problem is. You are the power in your house. I'll show you how to keep your own vibration up, and then even the lowest vibrating house *must rise to meet you.*"

* * * * * * * *

Thoughts And Emotions Must Agree

To manifest successfully, your thoughts and emotions must agree. Yes, it's possible to think something and have it appear—*if your emotions agree with your thought*. If your emotions don't agree, your energy is split. Think of emotions as valuable messengers that alert you to what you're really pulsing.

Emotions are too often feared and fled rather than valued and prized for the wisdom and power they offer. Forget public speaking, heights, and death—feelings are the most feared experience on the planet. Yes, some people do manage to get through *Things Are Going Great In My Absence* with some resistance, blind spots, and numbness still intact. If you still don't believe the Divine Openings mantra, "All feelings are good," intend now to get there, because it's vital to mastering your power of intention, as well as navigating your life.

We come here from the Non-Physical to revel in this sensory feast, and yet when the feelings get intense, we sometimes run from them, resist them, argue with them, blame other people for causing them, or try to do a spiritual bypass on them. A spiritual bypass is when you gloss over feelings, deny them, run from them, or explain them away with spiritual talk.

I've seen people resist feeling and look for loopholes to escape feelings for years before they finally appreciate them as the greatest treasure of all. If you've been numb to some of your feelings for a long time, it can take even Divine Openings a while to melt through that resistance unless you commit and *intend to feel fully*.

Once you appreciate all feelings, the lower ones will rise faster because you're no longer making them wrong. You get the payoff you really wanted—to feel better like your Large Self always does—relatively quickly.

Lower feelings alert you to reclaim the power tied up in them.

Rest and assimilate.

* * * * * * * *

Counter-Intentions

The number one reason intentions don't materialize is that intentions, energy, thoughts, or emotions are not all lining up and agreeing. We'll call it having counter-intentions: intentions that are split. You think you want one thing, but you actually want two contradictory things. For example: a person says she wants to claim her power, but she avoids going deep inside because intense feelings that she's run from all her life arise at first (that would end if she dived in and embraced them.) So she's constantly seeking, trying to find some new spiritual-bypass so she doesn't have to face her feelings by herself.

Of course that isn't working because by not feeling everything she's flying blind with no Instrument Panel and she hasn't learned to drive, so she remains mystified that she hasn't reached the mastery she's intending. Her counter-intention to avoid feelings is actually stronger than her stated intention of mastery.

Another example: A man's job of three decades became obsolete due to outsourcing to China. His stated intention was a new career, but he didn't realize he had a strong counter-intention to be right about how wrong outsourcing is. He was vibrating as an "innocent victim" of today's work world and the economy, and if he got a new job, to him it would unconsciously make it all OK that "his job was stolen by China." He didn't attract a job no matter how hard he worked at it. Once he let that go and got focused on where he wanted to go, he created a new career he actually enjoys more.

Counter-intentions split your energy, causing your desired outcome to be diminished, delayed, or never happen at all. Once you see what you're actually intending and beaming out there, you get a chance to clean it up.

With counter-intentions, you actually want two *apparently contradictory* things. The thoughts, intentions, and emotions are pulling in opposite directions instead of together, in integrity.

The counter-intention may not be obvious at first. You might *think* you want something with all your heart, but as you *feel* into it you might find out your desire is not wholehearted at all—there's a strong pull toward something else!

Here are some common counter-intentions:

- Intend to move, but want to stay where you are.
- Intend to commit (to a path, lover, project) but don't want to commit.
- Think you want adventure, but cling to security and stability.
- Feel love, but the mind is saying, "avoid getting hurt at all costs."
- Want change, yet want to stay in your comfort zone.
- Intend to find a better relationship, but want to maintain emotional or financial security.
- Intend a more expanded truth, but not willing to let go of old long-held beliefs or New Age clichés your friends believe in.
- Want to be your real self, but are worried if people will approve.
- Intend enlightenment, but also want to do what your seeker friends do.
- Want to create more money, but don't want to do new, challenging, or unfamiliar things to get it.
- Intend to create more money, but believe it will destroy your happy balanced life.

Counter-intentions are not necessarily bad—the intention and the counter-intention might be equally good, but just contradictory. I had two great but *apparently conflicting* intentions when my obsession to finish this book got in the way of my previous intention to take excellent care of my body. Once I consciously balanced the two I was able to have both. The exercise and good food actually *supported* the efficient writing of the book by increasing energy and vitality, and reducing the stiffness of sitting too long.

The point is to get your intentions clear, because all split intentions contradict, cloud, and dilute your power of intention. When your intentions are mixed, as you've noticed, your results are mixed.

Even if you choose to go with a counter-intention, at least you get relief and can stop fighting yourself. You can say, "I'm choosing this because it's safe."

Divine Forces immediately fulfill your desires, but conscious or unconscious counter-intentions like doubt, stress, disbelief, tension, or worry can delay it. There's no need to fix it or work on it. You're simply going to get clear and live more as your Large Self—then it all works out just fine.

An un-contradicted intention is a clear and potent intention.

Get Clear And BAM!

Clarify your intentions, and your power of intention grows without effort.

You might think you're purely intending to get a raise, and you're puzzled why it's not happening. Then you notice you have a strong counter-intention to prove your boss is wrong. You can't vibrate that your boss is wrong and get her to give you a raise, no matter how hard you work. You'll have to choose what you really want.

It's hard to find a great partner who won't bring you more disappointment while vibrating disappointment about past relationships, no matter how much you date or how many relationship techniques your learn. If you have a strong counter-intention that only bad people get rich and good people don't care about money, you repel money or can't hold onto it.

If you vibrate unworthiness, aware of it or not, it's hard to let good things in, or if you do let them in they tend to disappear. If you vibrate "victim," you get abused. If you vibrate anger, even if you try to squelch it or hide it under a nice, spiritual, and happy mask, you can still attract angry people, accidents, violent incidents, or inflamed or burning physical conditions.

Screeching just does not soothe a baby to sleep. A sleepy piano tune does not get people up dancing. Those vibrations just don't match up.

Grace and the goodness of Life weigh in on your side, but can't completely override your vibration. If your energy is split, your desired outcome can still happen, but it will take longer unless you shift. If part of you thinks it's possible, and part of you doubts it, your vibration is split. You're out of alignment with your Large Self, which always sees only unlimited possibilities.

Welcome to the human race. I catch myself in split intentions. I might want something to happen, but I'm so focused on what I don't like, how hard it is, or not having time to do it, I'm the source of the problem. You could call these misguided intentions, negative intentions, or back door intentions. I think each term adds clarity to the concept.

When I let go, what I want sometimes shows up overnight. I wanted my credit card company to do a better job with customer service, but the constant awareness of how poorly they were doing it created a counter-intention that slowed down the process. Finally I gave up, did some research, and got a new credit card with a company that gives twice the bonus miles, and then only later found out there was an added bonus: they win awards for their customer service! All I needed to do was focus on what I wanted, and stop focusing on the old company.

In one romantic situation, I'd tried communicating some desires, but I had an emotional charge on it and the person's resistance just increased. Finally, I dropped all focus on what he wasn't doing, withdrew my energy (but not my love) so abruptly he must have heard it snap. I skipped to the payoff and redirected my focus to "my ideal lover," relishing the *feelings I wanted* like they were happening right now. I spent a few minutes smiling at my new inner visions and went out and had fun.

There was a dramatic shift within two hours, and the things he said and did were so different than before (in a good way) it made my jaw drop. I won't tell you who that was. It doesn't matter. You can't lose—either the current person or situation will shift, or someone or something else will appear. Sometimes life is a progression of better, and better, and better.

ACTIVITY: Witness Any Counter-Intentions.

Jot down a few things you've intended to be, do, or have that have eluded you. Next to each one, write what counter-intentions you'd have to have in order to keep it from you.

1.

2.

3.

4.

5.

You're a powerful Conscious Creator! There's nothing to work on. Just consciously choose what to intend and what to let go of.

* * * * * * * *

Feel And Follow

When I'm riding my horse, if another horse shies at something, my horse might jump too; if there's a threat, he wants to know about it. When another horse runs, he wants to run too. He doesn't want to be left alone outside the herd. He'd run right into danger if the other horse did. We humans are herd animals too—fortunate in that we help each other, but unfortunate when we are compelled to do what others do even when it isn't working.

I created Divine Openings without need for validation or support from anyone, and for a while I was alone in it, but others did soon coalesce around me, and then that accelerated. There was no template or plan to follow—it was new, and there was trial and error, even with the strong guidance.

If you wanted rules, guarantees, unchanging dogma, or black and white answers I wouldn't give you those even if I thought they existed—I want you to feel in the moment and know from within.

Truth is relative to the circumstance, the time, the place, and your state of consciousness, and there is up-to-the-minute truth available to you at all times.

Divine Openings taps you into Pure Source, and your answers are always timely, current, fresh, and tailored for you—not for someone else, or some person who lived thousands of years ago. Life has evolved dramatically since then.

To claim your greatest power, ignore the herd.

Can you stay true to your intentions and heart's desires without support or validation from anyone? I do. I still don't need the support and validation I get, because I get it from within, and I give it to myself so powerfully. Give it to yourself first. I call this "being there for yourself." When you are there for yourself, others flock to join you.

Let go of any ideas you've picked up from media and other people that define for you the ideal community, city, country, partner, job, house, kids, life, looks, possessions, vacations, and hobbies. Instead feel little by little into your true heart's desires, giving them time to blossom in a way that's unique to you. It just might surprise you.

I'm even going to suggest that you may not know what forms would be best for you—that your Large Self knows, and would happily bring it if you'd let go of struggling for what the limited mind is set on.

A mere two years ago I was convinced I would *not* move out of Austin, but as soon as life steered me in the direction of California the energy of Austin felt old and dried up for me and I thought I'd pop if my Austin home didn't sell faster. Moving to California opened up a whole new world for me, and now I can't imagine it any other way. I've not missed Texas at all, and all my friends come to visit.

Fortunately I was so clear about the *feeling* I wanted that I was willing to let go and be flexible about the place, the physical forms, facts, and details of my new life. I could *feel* this change was right for me.

We don't always know what form would be best for us,
but our Large Self guides us to it.

ACTIVITY: Write down three *feelings* it's most important for you to feel in each area of your life. Of course they're not the only three feelings you want, but they're the most fulfilling ones in that department.

Your counter-intentions will emerge as well, alerting you to what's in the way, which ones you don't believe you can have, etc. Appreciate that they're making themselves known. Note them and you'll get clear.

Intended Feelings: Counter-intentions:

Work –

Play or leisure time –

Love –

Friendships –

Domestic situation or family –

Creative expression –

Contribution to others –

Mental stimulation –

Health –

Time –

Other areas of your life -

You can expect to get the *vibrational equivalent* of these feelings, although not always exactly the literal forms you think you must have. Let the forms surprise you. As long as you get the feeling you wanted, you'll be more than satisfied—you'll be deeply fulfilled.

For example, you might intend to get a job that makes you rich, but you actually get a job that gives you the feelings you thought only money could give you. Crucial point: appreciate it—you have the essential feeling you wanted—and the more you appreciate what you created, the more good will come.

You intend to find the perfect lover, but an unconditionally loving pet comes to you first, because you're not yet ready to let in human love due to some counter-intention like fear of getting hurt or being taken advantage of. Crucial point: You have the feeling you wanted. Fully appreciate the pet rather than making it wrong or not enough—and more love follows.

Specific superficial qualities may indeed not fulfill your true desires. Rather than writing down the specific qualities of your ideal partner, or how you want your spouse to start being, or where you want your new house to be, start general, with the feelings you want, which forms the matrix.

If what we want doesn't serve our evolution or meet our true heart's desires, our Large Self will try to steer us another direction. For example, having a lot of money may not serve some people. One man came into to a lot of money, but it didn't serve his spiritual development—he used it to buy his way out of situations rather than feel through them, stunting his evolution. Things always work out if we let them, though. He took a different path, and is now happily evolving.

* * * * * * * *

Stop Pushing Rocks Up Hills

In giving counseling, I'd been using the example of trying to push a rock up a hill to illustrate what it's like to try to do things all by human effort and physical means. When there was a big heavy metaphorical rock in some area of their life—maybe it was money or health or relationship or depression—they could feel the futility of trying to push that rock up that hill. They were ready for another way.

In the ancient Greek myth a man named Sisyphus was doomed to push a rock up a hill, only to watch it roll back down each time, for eternity. Sometimes you might feel like Sisyphus pushing that rock up that hill over and over.

The rock is down in a low spot with hills all around it, and every direction you could push it out of your way is *uphill*. You try, though. You strain and stress and manipulate and strategize. But it rolls back down after moving only an inch or two, if it moves at all. It feels impossible to move that rock, and it might well be impossible by physical human means only.

Other people you're not in control of might be your giant rock. Physical world limitations might be your rock. You're determined, though, and you give it everything you've got for as long as you can, but it's hard and never-ending, and you get exhausted.

It doesn't have to be that hard. Rather than coming up with better ways to push rocks or get stronger, we'll actually take the focus completely off the rock, and focus on your Non-Physical Self first.

Your small self is narrowly focused only on your physical being and your Earth life. It's limited, and sees fewer possibilities, excluding many of them as impossible.

From this Larger You, using all the Non-Physical power that's available to you above and beyond your human physical resources, there's a much easier way to move that rock without even trying to push it up the hill. As your Large Self, you vibrate what you want instead of paying so much attention to the problematic rock. Your Large Self isn't worried about the rock at all.

Your Non-Physical Large Self is everywhere, everything, and an unlimited array of possibilities are available, including things that don't exist yet. The difference in focus and perspective is enormous. To your Large, Non-Physical Self, moving a mere rock is a relatively small thing. When you're being your smaller, more limited self, moving a big rock is a very large and possibly insurmountable task.

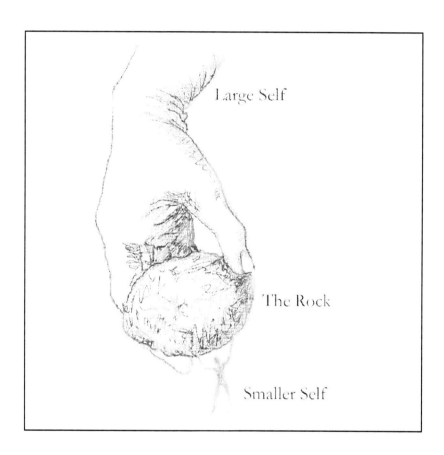

The relative power your limited self and your Large Self exert over the rock.

Pushing the rock uphill is the hard way. You can go straight to the Non-Physical source, where you constructed the rock, and construct something different—the easy way.

Focus on the *feeling* you think getting rid of the rock will give you, which creates an entirely new matrix to be physically filled in. Now you're vibrating very differently than you did when you materialized the rock. No need to exhaust yourself trying to push the rock up the hill. You sit, smiling quietly, or you take actions you're guided to take. Mostly you forget about the rock and have a good time.

ACTIVITY: How will you feel? Write in your notebook or the blank pages at the end of this book:

- How will you *feel* when the rock is moved?
- What will this new feeling inspire you to do?
- How will your world *feel* different?
- How much energy will you have when the energy tied up in moving the rock is recovered?

Once your vibration is consistently high about the rock and you're more focused on how you want *to feel*, the rock will move.

When I first wrote about pushing rocks up hills in a newsletter, Angeline Morrison, a graduate of the Five Day Silent Retreat who's a singer and an art professor in the United Kingdom responded with this brilliant bit:

> Dearest Lola, I'm really excited about the new book you're writing—your description made my mind whirl on all the possible ways the rock could move. A monster hovers in the skies above, raging and breathing fire. He suddenly sees the rock he was looking for! Smiling like a baby full of milk, he picks up the rock and flies away, cuddling it like a teddy bear and sucking his thumb.
>
> A man in a skintight pink jumpsuit and goggles walks up with a can of paint and a brush. "Step aside Miss, I'm sent by the Government Bureau Of Obstacle Removal," he says. He whistles a jaunty little tune as he paints over the rock with magical invisible paint. You watch, helpless with laughter, as it disappears.
>
> The rock turns into a beautifully wrapped birthday present, just for you!
>
> As it turns out, the rock is packed full of gold, diamonds and other riches. It's yours, so you get to sell it to the highest bidder.
>
> A gigantic fluffy kitten comes and pats the rock away, like a cat toy."

Angeline continues: "I actually can't stop thinking about that freakin' rock — it's taken over my mind for the time being, but what fun!

You never actually touched the rock, but you're overcome with curiosity and just have to poke it. As it morphs slightly, flattening itself, you discover it's a high-grade feather-stuffed mattress. You climb on for a little lie-down—but what's that humming sound? A thousand jewel-colored butterflies come carrying a feather quilt, and wrap you up softly for the most beautiful, dream-filled sleep of your life.

What's that young guy in a tracksuit doing over by the rock? Ah, he's a graffiti artist—he's tagging. You watch in amazement as he sprays and draws, creating amazing swirls and patterns and words. He's joined by more and more graffiti artists—it turns out your rock is the perfect canvas. More and more arrive, someone brings decks and starts DJ'ing. Still others bring food and drink and set up stalls. You can smell fried chicken and rice and cakes and hot chocolate and rum punch and all sorts of scents in the air, the beats are thumping, everyone's having a ball. All of it courtesy of your rock.

Of course, all of this can sound impossible and even terribly annoying if you haven't read *Things Are Going Great In My Absence* and ramped up your vibration prior to reading this book.

Notice how she engaged all her senses as she played creatively with the rock. We often dramatize our doubts, limitations and fears to rival a twenty million dollar Hollywood production, sparing no energetic expense—infusing our scary stories with Dolby sound and Technicolor in 3D. How often do we invest that much creative, sensory power and detail into *what we want to create?*

ACTIVITY: Stop and play with your "rock" from Large Self now. Make it mega-juicy!

* * * * * * * *

Creating Negative Intentions

When you spend your creative energy, time, and focus worrying, doubting, and feeling bad about what you lack, you're creating negative intentions. You're inking in a blueprint that the Universe will construct for you.

> *Your mind is a powerful instrument.*
> *Watch where you point that thing!*

Don't add resistance to resistance by fretting about your negativity. Once you dive into the feeling *and drop the story*, you are no longer creating anything unwanted—you're exempt. Negativity creates only when you're resisting feeling or hanging onto negative feelings, and going round and round in the story for some time.

If you can't yet dive in effectively, the link to get the Diving In Audios is: DivineOpenings.com/spiritual-enlightenment-audios. You might take the next online retreat, or get sessions. None of this is work—it's claiming your power—so working on "problems" will not get you there. This is *your life* we're talking about here! There is nothing more important.

* * * * * * * *

Balance Your Inner And Outer Life

Now we dive deeper into the Non-Physical. My words are intended to deepen your own access to direct knowing, not to install mere concepts. You deliberately intended yourself here to play in the physical realm. It's an exciting and challenging game at the leading edge of Creation, yet this physical realm is so engaging and distracting it's easy to forget it's not all there is of us and of life.

The smallest, most limited part of your reality—the physical—is the loudest, most tangible and intense for most humans. The Non-Physical impulses may be lost in the din of life, work, and busy activity—unless we regularly and consciously focus there.

We're attuned to the Non-Physical frequency when we're born, then as we immerse ourselves fully into this physical life, we adapt our tuning to the louder signal of this physical world and other humans. Most humans abandon their Non-Physical connection early in childhood, and some never find it again in this lifetime.

Once we experience awakening, we choose to tune back into the Larger reality of the Non-Physical and make it our main locus of power. Of course physical and Non-Physical is all One, and it will become more so once you find the balance, but keeping your focus on the Non-Physical opens you to your greatest power.

After feeling physically fabulous for a long stretch of time and being quite productive, for several days I woke feeling "off." My stomach was upset for no reason, and I had a slight, dull headache. I'd been writing madly on these two books, and enjoying it immensely. I'd just had a beautiful Sunday riding horses on the beach.

Sitting in front of a roaring fire in the hearth, I just surrendered to it, diving into the feelings underneath the physical distress as I stared blankly at the leaping flames. No story, no trying to figure it out.

Following that feeling led to a direct knowing: I have a peaceful life. I look out on mountains, trees, and nature. It's not a high-negative-stress life—it's a high-positive-stress life. I wake with ideas that spring me out of bed each day to do them. High frequency energy downloads come continually, and there's always more to do and write and create than I can keep up with.

My mind is active, although productive and positive most of the time. I'm busy creating, doing, writing, managing, counseling. And then I'm exercising, cleaning, arranging, going somewhere, socializing, riding horses, doing fun things.

In the stillness, the message was clear: it was time to stop and thoroughly digest all the incoming energy, allow it to assimilate in the stillness, with my mind at rest. Even channeling this high vibration writing wasn't pure rest. My body was telling me I needed to "just sit" and do absolutely nothing. "Don't be productive, don't go out and have fun, don't "do" anything!"

It felt wonderful to sit and blank my mind—deliberately thinking of nothing. I began the day with meditation instead of leaping out of bed ready to do things. Later, for fun I drove along with the radio off, intending my mind blank as I drove to do errands, strolled around the grocery store, and ate lunch. Usually I'll bring a book along on a solo lunch, and there's nothing wrong with that, but that day I savored my food and sat in The Void. That night I ended the day with meditation. I woke in the night with something that looked like wallpaper with green glowing daisies in a geometric pattern filling my field of vision. Ahhhhh.

Things get done for us in the quiet and stillness of the Fertile Void that we can't humanly fathom. The "me" that must take care of business in the world gets out of the way and rests while The Presence takes care of it. Many of you experienced being virtually "knocked out" while reading *Things Are Going Great In My Absence*. The Presence is saying, "Let me help you assimilate this before you go on, and it happens best with you out of the way."

This is why we don't try to duplicate the experience of the Five Day Silent Retreat in an online retreat. It just wouldn't be the same experience. We take care of everything for you for five days so massive realignment can happen with "you" and the distractions of your wonderfully juicy physical world out of the way. Then you can go live full out!

This is why reading (or even writing) spiritual books, getting counseling, taking courses, keeping your mind busy, learning new things, and constantly working on something actually distracts you from the very thing you say you're looking for. It's right there all the time—but it takes quality time and one-pointed focus to feel into it and experience it fully.

The stillness and quiet of The Void is restorative, so I gently dived into it until that energy was reclaimed, opening up luscious space.

If the physical world is avoided or neglected, your outer life can become a mess—your finances, relationships, health and body can stagnate or break down. Get out into the world more and take care of business. If inner focus is neglected, the Instrument Panel reads empty and disconnected regardless of outer world successes. Go within and experience the Source of you that is most real.

It makes me smile to feel the inner, then the outer pulling me in contrasting waves. Ooh, the physical world is so exciting I want to get out in it—I don't want to sit and meditate. Or, the silence and solitude is so luscious—I don't want to leave it!

Enjoy the gifts offered to you from both physical and
Non-Physical sources in balance.

The physical realm is key to evolution because the experiences it provides spur and spark our evolution. Every experience gives us new thoughts, new feelings, new desires—excites new possibilities—and our response to them drives movement in the entire Universe.

In the excellent HBO film Game Change, Ed Harris playing John McCain described how male role models in his life died or dried up once their reason to live disappeared. If work was their identity and meaning in life it's particularly common for men to die soon after retirement. When reasons to live disappear, energy doesn't flow; when energy stagnates, the body and mind stagnate. The entire physical Universe and even the Non-Physical realm need you to feed its movement and expansion.

You also need the contrast of stillness and silence to rest and restore yourself. By contrast each enhances the other. Please don't see contrast as "something wrong." Contrast is the variety that gives meaning and energy to its opposite. Think of contrast as a tasty menu from which you can choose.

Inner/outer

Stillness/movement

Silence/sound

Fullness/emptiness

Black or solid/White or blank

Light/dark

Lively/calm

Analytical mind/intuition and direct knowing

Action/rest

As I wrote this book, I'd take breaks to ride my horse, or lie in the sun on the deck looking at the trees to assimilate what I'd written, balance, and ground myself. I've needed a lot more solitude. Washing dishes or doing yard work grounds me and provides contrast. You're a vast Larger Being in the bigger picture, but in this more narrowly focused human life you're also a physical being trying to keep up with rapid expansion in this time of great acceleration. Take care of yourself as you would a precious child.

Go out and play in the big, wide, wonderful world you came here to experience. Intend what you want, and participate in the unfolding. Luxuriate in love and community, work and play. Then rest, clean off your hard drive, and reboot yourself in the silence. If you'll feel it and surf it, the contrast ultimately keeps you in balance.

Balance your inner and outer life moment to moment.

* * * * * * * *

How Does Intention Create?

Participants at the Five Day Silent Retreat laugh when I say at the end, "Your friends will ask, 'What did you do?' and you'll say, 'Nothing.' They'll ask, 'What did Lola give you or do to you?' and you'll reply, 'Nothing.' That'll drive them crazy and they'll push on, 'Well then, *what did you get?!?*'"

"Nothing."

Nothing" is an apt name for God.

You are created *from Nothing,* and Divine Openings helps you create *from Nothing,* just as the Supreme Creator does.

The deep, mysterious, Fertile Void is a Non-Physical non-place that I think of as the womb of Creation – the "nothingness" from which everything comes, and to which everything returns. In deep, ecstatic meditation or after Divine Openings, you've visited this silent empty space between your thoughts.

The Fertile Void is the Non-Physical, pre-manifest soup of all possibility and all potential.

This ineffable God we talk about is Everything *and* Nothing—and creates Everything *from* Nothing.

It is pre-energy and pre-vibration.

It is unlimited potential, manifest and un-manifest.

As we identify ourselves more with our Non-Physical being-ness we have increased access to our unlimited power, freedom, and joy.

Identify first and foremost with your Non-Physical Beingness.

You are God made manifest—God in physical form. Maybe you've heard this a thousand times, but have you actually let it in? Are you living it? It's not something to understand it and figure out, but to experience.

While Divine Openings and the power of intention really have nothing to do with gender, I find a gender analogy helpful just in this one context: When your intention—"male," active, dynamic thought energy, penetrates the Fertile Void—the "feminine", the mysterious, ineffable womb of creation, infinite possibilities and potentials are sorted and collapsed into synchronistic alignment with your intention. Your creation is fertilized on the Non-Physical level. Once it's ready to materialize, your creation emerges physically into this dimension.

There is no mechanism—it literally comes from Nothing, by pure intention. It's that easy. Really.

Intend as lightly as the touch of a gnat's wing. Let go and let The Divine do the heavy lifting. When you're guided to act, act.

* * * * * * * *

Resistance Is Your Friend!

Really. I mean it. I'm not kidding.

People sometimes panic about their resistance, wanting to get rid of it. They make it a bad thing, which not only adds resistance to resistance—it rejects a gift. Soothe yourself and don't give resistance any focus, because, yes, you guessed it, the more attention you give it the bigger it grows. Resisting our resistance feeds it energy and attention.

It's easier to let go of resistance if you *make the resistance right*. Make all lower Instrument Panel readings *right,* and then you can get their message. Make it right that humans disagree and have things to smooth out, since we all want something different. When you make it wrong, you're resisting that you live in a world of Free Will creators who all have different ideas.

Back when I led corporate conflict management courses, I'd walk up to someone and ask them to raise their hand with their palm facing me. I'd push my palm hard against theirs. They always pushed back! No one gave in, even the meekest person in the room! I'd ask, "Why are you pushing on my hand?" and the answer was *always,* "Because you were pushing *me.*"

Try this on: you actually enjoy pushing. You enjoy pushing yourself, other people, your limits, the limits of possibility itself; you find it stimulating and expanding.

Try this on: you like solving problems. You relish pushing against them, outwitting, or overcoming them. If you didn't have any problems, you would create some to have a challenge to resolve. When you work out with weights, you lift heavy objects to get stronger, and you do the same in life. It's true that sometimes we work *too* hard at it, but challenge does strengthen you and make you smarter. Evolution uses it.

Research shows that continuing to challenge your mind with new puzzles, learning, and challenge keeps you young and vital. Settle in, get soft, and stop growing, and you age faster.

Resistance is your friend.

Make resistance right. Soften into it, breathe through it, appreciate it, dance with it, laugh at it, embrace it, and allow it as part of your precious humanity. I see people fear it, fight it, talk about it, make it wrong, and work to release it, and it gets even stronger. We never ran out of issues when we focused on those and we never run out of resistances if we make fixing them our goal—that is the old fix-it paradigm, and it's endless!

Put your attention on how you want to feel and where you want to go, then gently and calmly feel the feelings that arise—resistant or not, they're valuable. Now we play with some ways to appreciate and benefit from resistance.

* * * * * * * *

Go Ahead, Draw Back The Bow

One day, as often happens, I was delighted to hear myself advising a client to think of her resistance as something that helps her build up potential momentum, much like you build tension when you pull the string back on a bow while aiming the arrow at your target. You're increasing the power and velocity at which the arrow will fly.

As you resist harder, as you pull back the bow but still do not let the arrow fly, you are making it more and more inevitable you will have to let go and when you do, the arrow will fly even faster. Anytime you make something right you loosen its grip on you.

Making it wrong is resisting your resistance! Make resistance your friend and appreciate it—for it tells you right where the difficulty is and increases the pressure to find a solution or let go.

Sometimes when I come up against a big challenge I have to stew in it for a while: "I don't like this. I *really don't like this.* That is wrong, and *that* is wrong, and *that must change!*" But after a while I'm done with that and I use the built-up tension to catapult me into a new place where I get focused on what I do want. It becomes an opportunity, which makes it right. I create a new matrix, and it all shifts.

Coming up from the back of the pack energizes some racehorses, like the famous champion Seabiscuit. If he started out in front, he didn't care if other horses passed him—he was such a smart character, in his mind he'd probably already won at the start, and quickly lost his motivation thinking about a nap and meal instead of the race. His trainer finally understood this and instructed the jockey to hold Seabiscuit back in the early part of every race, *resisting* his desire to run until he got jazzed up enough to win. The tension of being held back—the contrast of not being in the lead—brought out his very best and increased his desire.

There are times when you find yourself in resistance and it's tough to soften. Don't worry, resistance has its own way of working on you—it feels bad, which encourages you to shift. It helps you move. Resist a while. See how that removes resistance to resistance? Kinda makes you mad, too, doesn't it? That works, too!

Don't resist your resistance.

Anytime you embrace something and make it right, you reclaim power from it, alchemically raising its vibration to a powerful frequency you can use. Once you remove the resistance by making it right, it softens right then and there. Make it wrong and you tense up more.

It doesn't matter if you feel you're "making it up." You're making it all up anyway, so you might as well make up things that soothe and empower you. It's true because it works. Declare your resistance right.

Make resistance right and it softens.

Leading-edge innovators often address needs and problems before the public is ready to accept the improvements. The makers of electric cars are finding people aren't eager for such a big paradigm shift. When gas prices get painful enough, people will *demand* cars that don't burn fossil fuels. Some experts predict it will take ten-dollar-a-gallon gas to draw that bow back enough to sway the masses. Healthy, unprocessed food was resisted and called flaky for decades until diseases drew back the bow.

Resistance does its work one way or another.

ACTIVITY: Micro-Tensing

Micro-tensing uses conscious tension to release resistance. If there's a tight spot in your body, it began with a lower vibration that wasn't heeded, so it escalated and began to manifest itself physically. That area is crying out for energy that's pinched off by the tension of resistance. Rather than making it wrong, go with it and use it.

To play with micro-tensing, very, very slightly tighten the area that's already tight, so slightly that no one would notice you're doing it. Do it gently, light as the touch of a gnat's wing. That's why I call it micro-tensing—it's very small. Use your intention more than your muscles. By getting your body involved, you get out of your head, and *feel your intention* more tangibly.

Micro-tense that spot with your intention. Hold the tension a few seconds, then let go and relax into the relief, appreciating it, becoming more conscious of your ability to choose *tension* or *relief*. Play with a few more repetitions—prove to yourself that you have the choice to relax.

Resistance works for you if you embrace and value it! Resistance doesn't feel good, it's not supposed to, and eventually, eventually, eventually you'll let go.

That's my story and I'm sticking to it.

* * * * * * * *

Bounce Off What You Don't Want

Did you ever see one of those battery-operated toy cars that run in a straight line until they bump into something, then quickly pivot and go another way? They never stop and worry about the resistance of the wall. They never make the wall wrong—they just bounce off it.

They don't stop and study the problem—they just keep going. Like that little car, noticing what you don't want helps you redirect your intention toward another option. Just don't focus on the obstacle for too long. The trick is, quickly as you can, bounce your energy off that obstacle and head for the open road.

If your mind offers limitations for you, decline the invitation to play that game. Because "everyone does it," it might seem normal to focus on limitations. The limitation might even be "true"—you can see the wall, feel it, get validation from others to *prove it's there and that it's wrong*—but that would be giving it your power, and giving it even *more reality*.

Admit you don't want something, but quickly bounce off it toward what you do want. Bounce off thoughts, feelings, incidents, beliefs—anything you don't want—as you thank them for making themselves known to you and for propelling you forward.

For example, Tina's business partner was not carrying his weight anymore. Because of personal problems that he wasn't doing anything about, his attitude was sour. Tina tried the usual supportive, appreciative communication. She began to get angry when it wasn't working and she felt held back, but she used that anger as fuel. As soon as she declared that even if he didn't change it could be a blessing in disguise, that blessing began to unfold.

She began imagining how great she'd feel when she had a terrific team, people who loved their work as much as she did, and how great it would feel to cheerfully, creatively, and efficiently get things done. That created a whole new matrix that felt good now, and she knew it would flesh out into some kind of new reality.

When guided to, Tina again took the uncomfortable action of speaking to her partner, but the partner was defensive and uncooperative, so she let it go again. She kept her attention off the partner and on her new matrix, having no idea how it would all work out. A week later, after she prompted her partner to meet a crucial deadline, he started an argument and stormed out, saying, "I quit. You can buy me out and pay me off monthly over the next year." While relieved and exhilarated, there was still a touch of worry about how she'd get the all that work done *and* pay him, but she felt the feeling, dropped the story, shifted to feelings that would create the new matrix, and let go.

The next day a young man working in a coffee shop impressed her with his enthusiasm, warmth, energy, and intelligence. It turned out that he was working beneath his level just to make ends meet between big jobs; his skill set happened to be exactly what she needed, and he'd be willing to work his way up. She hired him after a short interview, and, along with an eager part-time retiree she hired, they all had fun, took the business to new heights, she easily paid off the absent partner, and now owns the whole, prosperous business herself—a blessing in disguise materialized.

No matter how frightening it looks at the moment, let that awful feeling bounce you off the obstacle and propel you in the direction you want to go. Sometimes people in a situation like Tina's will ask in a session, "What am I doing wrong? Am I creating this? Am I in resistance?" And I'll offer, "No, Life is just giving you a cue to change something. It's a blessing in disguise, one that's nudging you to move."

As you embrace that strong feeling of "I don't want this," making it right and looking for the blessing in disguise, that frequency rises up the Instrument Panel and becomes raw power you can use to make big, big changes. The moment you're clear what you don't want, it has served you all it possibly can.

Bounce off it as quickly as you can.

Every event, person, and speed bump, each turn, detour, and dead-end clarifies your desires as you recognize with humor and appreciation that you planted them there to nudge, irritate, prod, and lure you into further unfolding. You bounce off every solid wall you encounter, gaining velocity toward your desire in the process. Each fork in the road is an invitation to new possibilities.

You resist nothing, but use it all for your evolutionary progress. Now you're in the flow of Life, in harmony with All That Is, watching with amusement as the whole Universe begins to turn on its axis at your lightest intention to fill in your new matrix.

* * * * * * * *

Bounce Off The Bottom
If You're Down There Anyway . . .

We played with the idea of the little car that bounces off obstacles. Well, sometimes the little car falls in a hole. Some people give up after such a calamity and never reach in and pluck the car out. Others are actually energized by failure or challenge—it propels their desire to new heights. You get rubberized so if you drop you just "bounce off the bottom," never staying down for long. Better yet, though, the longer you do Divine Openings, the fewer holes you fall into—you usually feel them coming in plenty time to change course.

President Bill Clinton was dubbed "the Comeback Kid" because throughout his entire career he rebounded from impossibly bleak circumstances and obstacles others would have considered insurmountable, and still maintained unsinkable optimism. In fact, coming back after a loss seemed to energize him. The thrill of taking career-threatening risks certainly fueled his sexual escapades. I think he was one of our best presidents, and I have no judgments about the sex—but it was a career killing counter-intention, given the reality that the public always pays more attention to sex scandals than whether someone is doing a good job.

If you watch a news show and feel powerless, as if life is hard or unfair, or the government seems stupid or hopeless, bounce off it and stubbornly refuse to add any energy to that version of reality. Stop a moment, go within, breathe deep breaths, and deliberately focus on what you want.

Your intentions matter, and they really make a difference.

You can create the intention to bounce off the bottom anytime your vibration nosedives. Use the increased *oomph* that contrast provides to rev yourself up, choose another path, or try again with clearer intention. Make it a *productive* part of your story. "Contrast helps me feel more clear about where I'm going, and what I want and don't want." Once you start living into this, it becomes increasingly true for you.

When you jettison these stories you reclaim power:

- It matters what people think about me.
- I'll look bad if I stumble.
- I must be great from the start of an endeavor.
- People need to act differently for me to be happy
- Life is somehow wrong or unfair.
- The world is messed up and doomed.
- I need to fix the world or other people.

Notice that the above are out of your control or not your business. Don't waste your intentions and energy trying to control the uncontrollable—it just makes you tired. Stick to what you can do, apply your power where it counts. Handle your vibration, and it let it ripple out to the whole world.

More stories to let go of:

- Failure means something about me.
- Contrast is punishment.

- There's some end destination I must get to.
- There's something wrong with me. I'm flawed.
- I'm on earth, or that incident happened, so I'd "learn lessons."
- Karma, negative energy from someone else, the alignment of the stars, bad feng shui, or numerology is holding me back.

Claim you created it, no matter what. Use failures to bounce higher. It all works out.

Failure is merely a story, an interpretation of events.
Bounce off the bottom to new heights.

* * * * * * * *

Surf It

The mind wants to call what you're dealing with an issue or a problem, but that old paradigm gives difficulties, delays, problems, and challenges reality, weight, and seriousness they don't deserve. If you don't label something an *issue,* but call it *a feeling,* and *surf it* like a wave, resistance is reduced. Surfers don't call waves issues—they call them *fun!*

If you've been grappling with a feeling or challenge for a long time, call it a *vibrational habit* rather than an issue. Makes it softer, doesn't it? A vibrational habit can rise in frequency today if you just embrace it rather than making it wrong. There's nothing to clear, fix, or heal, and you're more empowered each time you let go of an old vibrational habit.

If you feel less than great, it just means your Instrument Panel is working. There's nothing to clear, fix, or heal. When someone tells me they need to clear this energy, emotion, or issue in their life, I'll say, "I think what you really want is to learn to navigate feelings, not get rid of them. You want to learn to surf your feelings so you can raise your own vibration anytime, anywhere."

I've watched surfers a lot, and they spend *most* of their time paddling out, waiting for waves, and falling off their board—all day long. They're in the troughs as well as on the crests—and it's not all glamour! They surf it all for the thrill of those moments when they are completely in the flow.

Surf it all.

* * * * * * * *

ACTIVITY: Choose Your Story Wisely

Your story either empowers or disempowers you, whether you know it or not, and you will live that story. The story you tell expresses an intention. Feel your body as you tell each story. Which feels better?

- It's not fair that I'm being taken advantage of.
- This is giving me fuel to make a powerful change. I'm bouncing of it to go higher.
- The economy is down, and it's greedy rich people's fault.
- I create my own economy. I let The Divine do the heavy lifting and send waves to carry me. I'm surfing it all.

As I say in my song collection, *Watch Where You Point That Thing*, "Your mind is a powerful instrument. Watch where you point that thing." It's available at DivineOpenings.com and spans from dance to meditation music. Click Divine Music in the menu.

Appreciation Increases Power Of Intention

Some of you have already become "automatic appreciation generators," and your power is awesome. Lets expand it out even further.

Appreciate for a moment all of the Non-Physical forces that are focused on your happiness and success right now. Feel how they take joy in arranging, orchestrating, lining up and preparing things for you. They're sending you signals and signs, sending people to intersect with you, or even making you laugh. It's as if you have a team of managers, assistants, facilitators, healers, geniuses, and specialists in any area you need. All you have to do is let it in.

Even Non-Physical beings love appreciation, although they don't relate to having names and identities like we do. They're not separate from us at all, and they're not somewhere else—they're right here, right now. Appreciate that your Large Self is One with everyone dear to you who ever passed on from the earth plane, and others you haven't met yet in the physical. I experience all this as direct knowing that seems to come from nowhere, but occasionally can feel my deceased dad, grandmother, past teachers, and others. I often smile and say thank you when I get a hit of knowing out of nowhere. Many people tell me they experience my Non-Physical aspect visiting or helping them in this way, but it's not my human self.

Back to the physical, I *appreciate* the services and products I received as I pay bills. Wow, they give me electricity without a care! Water just comes out of my pipes! I got a home on credit without paying cash! After years of this, I've paid off all debts except for the house. When I move to a new home, the trees and bushes start growing very fast. They flourish because I appreciate them, gaze at them, and delight in how their leaves or flowers are growing. There's no ceremony in any of this, it's just a way of life.

Appreciation sets up a vibration at the same frequency as love, a very high vibration indeed. As you pulse at that frequency, you feel good—that alone is enough reason to do it. Keep your focus on the generation of good feelings so you don't reverse them fretting about anything that hasn't materialized yet.

I learned to appreciate and authentically embrace disagreement between strong, smart, opinionated people. With the focus on appreciation of disagreements rather than how unpleasant they are, resistance dissolves and disagreements feel better. Feeling better is everything.

Some of the smartest and even the most metaphysically educated people are among the unhappiest, because when the mind is in control, that wrong-seeking missile burns a lot of energy and intention going after everything that's wrong.

It might be smart to be in the know about what's going on in the world, but is it productive—really? Feel this. If we buy into reality as if we are mere passive observers, we abdicate our power to create reality. Match the vibration pinging from your Large Self and you create rather than observe. Yes, it can be challenging, but it's worth mastering.

You don't just observe reality—you create it.

Appreciation is choosing to focus on the good, which takes you where your Large Self is on every subject. It's finding a small shred of something you can appreciate amidst a pile of things you have difficulty appreciating. No doubt you've heard the funny story of two kids—one an optimist, the other a pessimist, and how they responded very differently to the same circumstances. The pessimist was told there was something for her in a glass observation room filled with horse poop. After only a minute, she came out angry and complaining about the stink and the pointlessness of it.

The optimistic child was sent in, and became *enthralled* with shoveling through the poop from one end of the room. When asked why she wouldn't come out, her enthusiastic reply was, "With all that horse poop, I figured there had to be a pony hidden in there somewhere, and if I didn't quit, I'd eventually find him."

Appreciate because it feels good. Appreciate to amp up your vibration. Most of all, appreciate before the goods arrive. *Skip to the payoff* and feel good now—assume there's a pony in there somewhere. Long before I got a pony at age nine, I was drawing ponies, adoring ponies, and reading books about ponies.

My intention was stubbornly, passionately powerful, and I stuck to it, while enjoying the feeling I got drawing ponies. My parents were living month-to-month, my dad supporting all five of us as he worked and went to night school, but somehow they found a way to get me that first pony, Star Baby, that in retrospect looked just like my drawings. Decades later, I got the ranch I had drawn in such detail so many times, with its pond and trees, house, truck, ducks, dogs, and horses. I always drew it from up in the air, from what now looks to me like Large Self big-picture perspective.

Do the best you can. Practice daily; choose your attitude by the minute. Rave about what's great when you wake and before you go to sleep, and over time you'll get addicted to how good it feels. As you tune your mind to the appreciation frequency, it becomes a vibrational habit. You amp up your power to create with intention by being one with your Large Self and your unlimited Non-Physical power.

Life is what you make of it. Always was. Always will be.
— Grandma Moses, the American folk artist who began
painting in her seventies (1860-1961)

ACTIVITY: Appreciate Right Now

Tag this page, and come back to it daily until this is a habit and you no longer need this reminder. Give yourself the daily pleasure of doing a combination of these. The more uplift you need, the longer you do it.

- Rave about twenty things you appreciate, no matter how small. (If you can't think of that many, *you need a lot more practice!*)
- Appreciate your Non-Physical team and the infinite help that's there for you.
- For the valuable Instrument Panel reading it gives you, appreciate a feeling you don't like. Feel your vibration rise from the appreciation of it.
- Appreciate an obstacle as you intend to bounce off it.
- Find something you can appreciate about someone you judge. Feel your energy increase.

It's not work. Do it often, *for fun*.

* * * * * * * *

You Go Where You Look

Have you ever noticed when you're driving along the highway and look at something off the road to your right, how you tend to veer to the right? If you're not careful, you could even run off the road.

You go where your nose is pointed.

During my life, I've vacillated between not allowing any mainstream media input into my happy life, and letting just selective bits in. It's always wise to be selective, but it's vitally important if you're still raising and/or stabilizing your vibration. Notice how you feel.

You might be already so unsinkable you can keep your vibration up in the face of negative input or find the beauty in anything, but if you're not quite there yet, don't ingest it. I just don't choose input that doesn't feel good, even if I can keep my vibration up. Most people who wouldn't even think of eating junk food think nothing of ingesting gossip, or negative news and entertainment.

The magazine *Fast Company* is fascinating to me because it focuses only on new-school, leading-edge creative and business innovators, not old-school thinking or the Wall Street mindset. It's about people who create trends rather than follow them. It helps me stay abreast of some of the best of what's happening in this fast-changing world and I pick and choose what's stimulating to my own creativity.

One recent in-depth article was about director Martin Scorsese and living a creative life. Scorsese has followed his own inner compass all along, which didn't always ingratiate him with the big Hollywood studios. Now older than most people are when they retire, he's only recently coming into esteem among Hollywood insiders with big budgets.

Interestingly, like Clint Eastwood and Woody Allen, Scorsese's heart has softened and he's no longer an angry man—he's doing more uplifting films now. His wife had commented, "Why don't you make a film our daughter can watch?" It was wonderful to watch him thank his twelve-year-old daughter as he accepted his Golden Globe Award for his film *Hugo*.

Woody Allen also won acclaim for his uncharacteristically uplifting and meaningful *Midnight In Paris*, a far cry from the nihilistic films with angst-ridden characters of the past. The message of the film is that "now is the perfect time to be alive." Some allow age to soften them—others just get more hardened.

Focus Is Like A Muscle

A large element of building your power of intention is to practice. If you want to build a muscle, you use it, even stress it, regularly. And yes, if you get lazy and unconscious, just like the muscle, your power of intention goes lax. You simply cannot go back to sleep and maintain your power of intention.

Inner/outer balance requires daily choice and focus. Fully, joyfully, enthusiastically engage in the physical world and play the game of Life On Earth, remembering the physical is only a small part of who you really are. Remember that what's going on physically right now is not the ultimate reality—it's a temporary reality—and you are a Conscious Creator. Witness yourself with compassion and let your Large Self guide you.

If you want a great life, be deliberate in how you think and where you focus. Catch yourself in less-than-productive thoughts before they carry you away. You have to think and make choices every day anyway—you might as well do it well and consciously, even *stubbornly*. If you think of yourself as stubborn or resistant, be stubborn about where you put your focus, what you believe, and what you want. Be stubbornly unwilling to settle for anything less than a high vibration and a wonderful life.

If you're a nurse, a doctor, or an accountant, decide today that your real job is to be clear and happy. If you're an attorney, a plumber, or a cook, make it your job to enjoy every single moment you can and leave every person you encounter uplifted.

Life offers you many choices. Direct your focus toward what supports you, and withdraw it from what doesn't support you.

Use your power of intention to embrace a liability and turn it into an asset. By embracing every feeling that arose during my move to California, they moved, and I was moved forward. By not making those lower feelings wrong or running to someone to get them fixed, each moment led to the next opening, the next bit of relief. Evolution works—Life is designed to move you.

While still in Texas, I began to feel and talk as if I'd already moved to California. *In the Non-Physical I already had moved*—I was just waiting for my body to catch up. I say this with a smile: don't let little things like your current physical reality influence you too much. It's temporary. Your current reality is already history.

You're not creating anything negative when you're deliberately and consciously being with lower feelings, so don't stress about it. You're in a state of Grace that literally exempts you from the Law Of Attraction when you're consciously feeling, with the intention to let go and soften. You only create something negative when you unconsciously vibrate low for some time, or are resisting feeling or change.

Drop the story about *why you have the feeling*, embrace the feeling itself, with no story whatsoever running in your head "about it." No words, no narrative, unless you need just a few key words to help you feel it fully. A woman told me just the other day that she thought she'd been doing the Diving In process from *Things Are Going Great In My Absence,* and it just wasn't working—then one day her Large Self got through to her and said, *"Stop! You're diving into the story, not the feeling!"*

Intention, Addiction And Food

Many wonderful things as well as those we think of as destructive can become addictive: work, new relationships, sex, drama, thrill-seeking, pornography, escapism, food, drugs, anti-depressants, pain killers, numbing out, smoking, alcohol, rage, gambling, risk-taking.

My definition of addiction is simple: it's a vibrational habit that is persistent but doesn't serve you, and it's hard to stop.

Here's how it works:

- One uses or does something (we'll call it a fix) to try to feel better.
- The relief is short term, so it must be done habitually.
- It becomes a *vibrational habit* that is self-perpetuating.
- A built-in rationalization system stubbornly justifies the habit.
- Soon it takes more of the fix to get the same relief.
- Eventually the fix gives *no* relief, but the vibrational habit persists.
- Addictions usurp our power of intention and commandeer Free Will.
- Getting relief ceases to be the intention, *getting the fix is now the overriding prime intention!*
- The bad feeling creates more desire to feel better, thus more fix.
- All addictions trade off long-term good for a short-term fix.

I do not consider addictive vibrational habits, even ones they call "serious" to be a big a deal as long as a person truly commits to regain his power. Everything is temporary. Life wants to move.

Like all of us, people who are addicted
are just trying to feel good.

Intend now: notice when you're using any fix to try to *feel better*, relieve pain, avoid feeling bad, relax, numb out, let go, feel loved, feel nurtured, or socialize. The deep emotional need is what really keeps one addicted to the fix—the physical part of the addiction is the weakest part. Stay off the fix for a few days and the physical craving diminishes quite quickly. The emotional need, though, will not just disappear—it requires filling.

What's the remedy for addictive vibrational habits?

- Make *feeling better* your prime intention.
- Feel the feeling you're trying to relieve—boredom, loneliness, doubt, anger, fear, sadness, grief, unworthiness, powerlessness?
- What do you want to feel? *Intend to generate that feeling.*
- Feel forward into the long-term good feeling you want, and ways to get it will appear.
- If it's energy you want, intend energy, move your body, dance, drink water, breathe slowly and deeply for five solid minutes.
- If it's love, intend love, get a pet, make friends, volunteer, fall in love, open your love pipes.
- If it's to fill a void, intend it filled in a healthy way, talk to The Presence, meditate, and get a life.
- Your Large Self already feels good, so when you go to Large Self vibration you feel good without the fix.
- Get sessions or rehab if you need help getting over the hump.

Focus on the long-term feeling you want rather than
reaching for a short-term fix.

Food and body weight are one area where people aren't as clear how intention and vibration work. Overnight you can get healed from a disease, fall back in love, or receive a pile of money—but weight doesn't change quite that quickly—you often don't see exciting results for months, so focusing on the long term is extra important.

Food addiction, using food as a fix to medicate feelings, is tricky, because food is the only addiction you can't stop cold turkey—you still have to eat three times a day. If eating is your favorite or only way to feel better, and you're not able to use your Free Will choice to find another way to feel better, *that is food addiction.* Because addictions have a powerful self-rationalizing mechanism, it takes commitment to be a Conscious Creator.

When you have counter-intentions, the one that feels the
best to you wins, even if it's only a short-term fix.

PRACTICE: Feel Better Without The Food Fix

Intend your lean, light, healthy, happy self now. Then virtually every time you want to put something in your mouth, very consciously and intentionally:

- Stop and feel whether you really *need fuel* or whether you just want a quick fix to feel better.
- Feel the feeling you're trying to relieve, drop the story, and dive in.
- Intend the feeling you *want* to feel.
- Find treats to give yourself that don't go in your mouth.
- As above, if it's energy you want, intend energy, move your body, dance, drink water, and breathe slowly and deeply for five solid minutes.
- If it's love, intend love, make love, open to love, get a pet, make friends, volunteer.
- If it's to fill a void, intend it filled in a healthy way, talk to The Presence, meditate for pleasure more often, get more of a life.
- Notice your fears and counter-intentions about choosing the healthier choices.

Choose other ways to feel better besides eating.

* * * * * * * *

People with a lot of extra fat have a low vibration in some area—maybe self-worth, feeling they need protection, over-giving to others, or generally sluggish emotional and physical energy. This is an observation from vast experience, not a judgment—people vibrating "victim" are almost always:

- Skinny, pinging the vibrational signal, "I am small and powerless."
- Overweight or out of shape, pinging the signal, "I'm trying to shield myself with fat, or numb or comfort myself with food."

But the feelings come from the inside—shielding the outside is futile. One woman wanted much more privacy and adult time than she was getting now that she had a son, and her body was trying to literally claim more space for her. She discovered this counter-intention: *to her body* the extra fat felt like protection. Of course her son wasn't really invading her—that was just the small self's perception and survival response.

The vibration wasn't very low, so her weight gain was just a few pounds. She talked soothingly to her body and assured it she would take care of it without the need for a fat shield, and massaged her vibration upward. She took better care of herself emotionally, took little trips with friends, was mindful not to take on family members' vibrations and emotions, or comfort or reward herself too much with food. She lost fat quickly.

When I was first diving into writing this book, I dropped everything else for a few weeks, including exercise and some really self-nurturing eating habits. I got sloppy about my food choices, and found myself hauling around a few extra pounds. Calling it post-menopausal body weight was a story that just made me feel powerless about it, and I started looking for lean older people everywhere I went—there are plenty, and that blew that story.

The conflicting intentions were my obsession to finish this book fast, and my intention to take care of my body. My body lost that contest for a while, and it soon complained loudly—it liked the previous lifestyle better!

I also realized I had defaulted into a social evening ritual of using rich food, a glass of wine, and sedentary pastimes as end-of-day treats. Wine and heavy food make me feel sluggish soon after consuming them and on the following morning, and the pounds can creep up. It's a very human intention to blend socially, even if it compromises our own wellbeing, but it's unlike me to succumb to anything that runs counter to sparkling clear consciousness.

Treats that signal the end of the workday and help us relax and play are enormously important. My intentions were health, to be light and lean and feel great, and to reward myself—but the quickest, easiest fix that worked socially wasn't working out. When I felt it and got clear, I wanted my prime intentions much more than I wanted any of the quick fixes.

If the body is accustomed to eating or drinking certain things, it takes a few days of withdrawal from the addictive habits to recalibrate the body's Instrument Panel. It wants *whatever* it's been getting, and insists on more of that *even if it no longer makes you feel good.*

If we've been telling our body that junk food is yummy, and vegetables are yucky, and we want it to think "vegetables taste good," we have to recalibrate the Instrument Panel—it's out of whack, upside down, and its readings are off. The very foundation of addiction is that the body wants whatever we've accustomed it to, whether it's good for us or not. Anyone can get the Instrument Panel messed up, but it's easy to get it working properly again.

At first, it was an effort to talk my system into changing its cravings, but once changed it I felt so good it was easy to maintain it. I found more creative ways to reward myself with walks, hikes, horse and bike rides, lighter evening meals, fresh juicing, sparkling water, movies, and massages. I intended friends to do more of these things with, and they appeared.

One way to ease transitions is to *add* healthier things *before* you subtract the less healthy ones. Add fresh home juicing and exercise first before you subtract the greasy food—that helps recalibrate the Instrument Panel by contrast.

Ingesting anything while feeling it's bad is *abusing yourself*—guilt takes you down the Instrument Panel. Eating well can give you a fabulous feeling of taking care of yourself—now that's the kind of emotional eating I like.

Notice when your intention for short-term relief is stronger than your intention for long-term relief, because the strongest intention *always wins.* Focus on and commit to your long-term intention.

Using everything I felt and experienced as feedback, I got better and better at it over time. Simply by getting more intentional about how I wanted to feel, slowing down, choosing wisely like I used to, and savoring food more, I was soon leaving food on my plate. That was new. I wasn't trying—my intention just started playing out that way. The counter-intentions can be reconciled. I'm back in balance, having it all. It's really about staying awake.

Feel your food choices and ask yourself, "What's going to feel good to my body right now AND feel good tomorrow? What's going to taste good now AND let me feel great about myself in a month?" I literally ask myself when faced with the sweet rolls and donuts at the pastry counter, "What do I want more, a fleeting five minute taste-bud treat, or to maintain the fantastic feeling of this light lean body?"

Nine times out of ten, I smile at how much I love this light, lean body, and walk away with just a coffee, or go home and stir up my own healthy chocolate that actually encourages a healthy metabolism. Using super foods, I make enough for a week in just five minutes. Melt together equal parts of raw cacao, raw honey, coconut oil, shredded coconut, and crushed nuts. Stir in a spoon of cinnamon and a dusting of cayenne and turmeric. Chill.

Focus on where you're going, not on what's wrong, because your Large Self is not with you in making it or you wrong. It's just a choice.

Don't focus on losing weight—intend to feel light and lean.

ACTIVITY: Intend To Choose How You Feel More Often
Intend how you want to feel about food. Walk yourself through this journey as you smile softly, read with soft eyes, and breathe in each sentence.

- Know yourself as God in a physical body.
- Intend to feel love for yourself and your body.
- Intend to meet your emotional needs with other things besides food.
- Start with eating foods you already feel good about and rave to increase the harmonious feeling while eating them.
- S-l-o-w d-o-w-n and savor the preparation and the eating.
- Intend good feelings about your food choices rather than focusing on weight loss or calories.
- Choose food by how it feels to your body *after* you eat it.
- Taking care of your body is an act of love.
- Notice your counter-intentions about food, and intend how you'll feel when there's no split energy.
- Feel the long-term feelings you want.

If someone vibrates, "I want to be lean," and "All the good foods make me fat," at the same time, those are obviously contradictory intentions.

There is no single truth about food or anything else I can package for you. I can't say this is good for you and that is bad for you. Truth shifts, depending on the reality you're in. It's all true in some reality. Higher consciousness is not about learning all the esoteric secrets and rules; it's being a Conscious Creator rather than looking for truth outside ourselves. Will we each master everything in this lifetime? Maybe, maybe not, but either way we'll have a fabulous life.

Truth is different in different realities.

Alcohol is poisonous for some people, yet can be completely benign for others. One famous spiritual master popped five tabs of LSD back in the Sixties to make a point for the hippies who were attracted to his high, light, free vibration. The acid had no effect on him whatsoever—he just laughed. Then to further his point, he radiated a blast of shakti that blissed everyone out. He was the most powerful component, not the drug. His Non-Physical power completely superseded his physical reality—very advanced, but it's possible.

I haven't jumped the body matrix and exempted myself from *all* the rules of physical reality quite yet, although I'm doing all right. I still eat healthily and exercise to keep the body fat down. But I jumped the collective money matrix a long time ago, making it a non-issue, and created a new relationship matrix quite recently. There's no set timetable, and everyone gets there when they do, and you can have a great life on your way there. I was having a great time surfing it all along.

I actually *adore* the feeling I get from eating lighter-feeling food and exercising. It makes me feel good—alive, strong, and vital. I don't like the feeling I get *after* eating heavy, rich food. The key thing is to do what *feels good now and later.*

Healers, counselors, mothers, enablers, and over-sensitive people can let other people's problems *weigh them down*—they're literally carrying too much heavy vibrational weight, and the body expresses it. If they have no idea they're doing it they might eat to shed stress, which makes it worse.

If you sponge up low vibrations from others, your body complains, "If you won't handle this vibrationally, I'll put up a fat shield. You leave me no choice." Fat piles on and won't come off until you stop sponging and take care of yourself.

Occupy all of your own energetic space, and you won't need to get fat to physically own your own space. Make your *energy* big. Even tiny people can command the attention of big, pushy horses, dogs, or people when they project big energy, and they instantly get more respect.

Healers and counselors can also put on weight if they believe in the need for psychic protection from negativity or dark energies. Using "spiritual protection methods" just pings out the message that you're a victim. That *attracts bad stuff,* reinforcing belief in the need for protection, which makes you feel like more of a victim and—see the spiral?

I've never seen anyone use spiritual protection who didn't create many, many negative things to protect herself from—the so-called protection doesn't even work. Just assume it's not needed—and be conscious about when you're taking on other people's energies or problems.

Twenty years ago I stopped giving any power to imaginary dark or evil forces after a terrifying evil presence woke me one night. Its face was two feet from mine, ugly, rotting, and menacing. My Large Self instantly told me, "It's a part of you." So I said to it, "Hello, old friend. I accept you, I welcome you home, I'm not afraid of you." It disappeared, along with the scary dreams I used to have, and nothing like that has ever happened again. It's all me. It's all you. Intend now to reclaim your power from fear of outside forces. There is no outside force.

You're sponging if you:

- Worry about others' problems.
- Try to help people who need to help themselves.
- Feel bad with them, sympathize, or empathize in ways that lower your vibration rather than bringing theirs up to yours.
- Stress about someone's struggles. Your Large Self never feels bad about them, but stays high, loves them, and sees their Large Self as capable and evolving, which helps them.
- Feel you need to use spiritual protection methods, which actually attract negativity due to believing in outside danger.
- Believe that anything that wasn't created vibrationally by you can harm you.
- Can't hold your own vibration high when you're in crowds, or feel you're too sensitive. This is not just sensitivity—it's victim vibration that allows your energy to be affected by others.

So what to do? There's an activity in a later section that helps you beam your energy out so powerfully that there's no room for unwanted energies to enter your energy field. Then the matrices you create are clear, clean, and *yours.*

Intend to know your power, walk your talk. Refuse to give any power away. Say, "I create it all." If you're still sponging, be extra careful who you're with and what you sponge up. Read about, emulate, and be with uplifting people you want to be like, who give no power away to anything. I'd never tell someone who was spiritual bypassing to just smile, but once you're in your power, just smiling can shift your vibration!

Smile, stay high, stay light.

Just as I find it puzzling that many people who go "spiritual" also go broke, I find it puzzling that many people who go "health-conscious" also get more afraid of food, and sometimes *less healthy!* The health food aisles are populated with a lot of worried, unhappy, unhealthy-looking people fervently studying labels, squinting beneath furrowed brows.

"It all has something in it that will kill you," and "Restricting my eating to certain foods is the only way," are common beliefs. I know—I've been there—I became a rabid health-nut at age sixteen, baffling my parents. In many ways this served me incredibly well—it helped me avoid all the hereditary diseases in my family and slowed the aging process. In other ways it limited me by giving food too much power.

There are plenty of well-meaning practitioners demonizing all kinds of foods and fostering fear of food, the environment, and all kinds of things. When you're clear, you can intuit, experiment, and benefit. When you're not clear you can give too much power away. When you become the most powerful component in the food equation, you can eat anything.

When people attend the Five Day Silent Retreat, their food allergies and sensitivities mysteriously disappear. We discovered this by accident. We used to try to accommodate people's dietary restrictions, but it became completely ridiculous—so many spiritual and illness-conscious people eat wildly varied diets, and each one is sure her diet is the only way and that she will suffer dire consequences if she don't follow it. Yes, we call that *illness-conscious*, not *health-conscious!* The dominant focus is on illness and fear. Attention quickly sneaks into becoming intention.

Is the intention really health consciousness—
or is it illness consciousness?

Logistically, we had to stop catering to diets and food austerities, and I didn't believe in them anyway, so I knew somehow it would work out because I create a powerful matrix that is the most powerful component at the retreats. The participants are enveloped in and attuned to such a powerful vibrational vortex that they align with it, and step into much Larger versions of themselves. Then something interesting happens. *Suddenly, food is not more powerful than they are.* They become the dominant component, not the food.

The retreat doesn't take away your Free Will, nor would we want it to, even for your own good, but people do go home fully equipped to maintain their elevated state. Most do, but a few are sloppy and fall back into the old vibrational habit of giving power away to food and other things once I'm not there holding the matrix in place any longer.

Responding like a victim to a harmless substance in the environment is exactly like running from scary things we create in our own dreams or visions. Fearing a perfectly normal food creates a harmful vibration, but it's not the food causing it, it's us.

Believe me, your Large Self doesn't have food allergies, or any other problem. Allergies are a mistaken defensive response to non-dangerous substances—always an indication of some kind of victim vibration. I had allergies, but the day I learned this thirty years ago, a gong literally rang in my head, and I never had allergies again.

True, there *are* realities in which people have all kinds of allergies and food sensitivities. All I'm saying is that when you claim more of your power as a Conscious Creator, it doesn't have to be *your* reality. Environmental sensitivities are real at one level of consciousness, yet they disappear at the level of consciousness where the person *feels* the world is a safe place to live.

What is the most powerful vibrational component,
you or the food?

Do live by the rules of the old reality if you're still in it. Do whatever you need to do to nurture that precious vehicle, your body, and feel good. Eat well, move, play more. At some point some of you will switch realities, and you will assimilate all foods better. Then, at the next level you don't have to be so concerned about what you eat. The rules shift with the consciousness. Don't strive or stress about this. Set your intention and enjoy life.

The desire to find absolute truth outside yourself can hobble you because there are so many *proven, validated, true* threats out there. If you buy the science and statistics, you give away your miracle-producing power. Science can prove that your disease is incurable, but a miracle can make your disease or allergy disappear.

It can upset our comfort zone to have reality bend and flex, since we really want to *depend on our reality to be reliable*. For example, I initiate people to heal physical disease, and then give them a chance to heal something really serious, such as leukemia or a traumatic injury, and they do it. Later, however, some have a backlash—their mind goes into resistance and tries to talk them out of believing they actually can do that, *even after they have done it*.

If you eat with the thought that a certain food is bad for you, it is indeed bad for you, because *your intention* creates resistance to it and causes your body to assimilate it poorly. If you make a food your enemy, you've set up vibrational disharmony with it, so if you eat it you will gain weight or have a bad reaction to it! Live by the rules of the reality you're in until you shift that reality.

Notice your *intentions* as you shop, prepare food, and eat. If your intention is protection from harm, you're increasing the vibration of fear, giving away power, and cancelling the benefit of the food. If you are vibrating that most foods are bad for you, you're creating disharmony between you and most of the foods in the store.

When someone is vibrating, "I want to be healthy," and "All the good-tasting foods are bad for me," those are big contradictory intentions. But notice that your counter-intention is actually not true—*it's a story*.

You've established a vibrational relationship with any foods you've made wrong, and if you're to ever eat them again and still be healthy and light, you'll need to change that relationship. If you're going to drink alcohol occasionally (but not to medicate, please) appreciate it and harmonize with it. If you feel guilt, that's low on the Instrument Panel, not up where your powerful Large Self vibrates, so drinking with guilt lowers your vibration. But not because the *substance* has the power to lower your vibration—only *you* have the power to do that.

So, you see, the food-Nazis are right, and the eat-it-all-in-moderation people are right, and some of the eat-anything people make it work too. You'll master the power of intention in some areas of your life faster than others. The more you relax, make all your feelings right, and simply accept that you are where you are now, the faster you'll go. Slower is faster with Divine Openings, and the best news is: you can be happy the entire trip, long before the physical result you think you must have arrives. I've relaxed into this so much that there's really not anything I'm longing for. Sure, I have some desires, but there's plenty of time; they're coming.

It's literally intending to harm your body to consume something while vibrating that it's harmful.

Some people bless their food before eating it, but I think you'll find the activity below clearer and more powerful: *you just line up with the food, and line it up with you.* It doesn't assume there's anything in the food or you that needs fixing. It's just a vibrational alignment, and creating by intention is all about alignment!

ACTIVITY: Harmonize With Your Food

Tag this page. Begin practicing with food you think is good for you. Next time you sit down to eat, slow down, take a big deep breath, and intend to enjoy and s-l-o-o-o-o-o-o-w-l-y savor your food.

Sitting tall, close your eyes, and smile into your stomach. Smile into the food, breathing harmony and agreement for three or four breaths.

Or, you can hold your palms toward the food and appreciate the food, which harmonizes with it. It's the intention that matters, not the ritual.

Set the intention that your body uses food efficiently and gets everything it needs. If you can't feel good about a particular food, don't eat it. Choose another.

You may do this for a while before you master it and become the most powerful component. Life's feedback and your feelings will guide you to recognize and let go of counter-intentions and limiting beliefs.

* * * * * * * *

Don't Forget To Graduate

You don't need training wheels once you can ride the bike. Once you've dialed the phone and the person has answered, you quit dialing and talk. Once you've met your soul mate, you quit dating and deepen and unfold the relationship. Unless people find great pleasure or joy in practices, most practices or processes are naturally outgrown.

You'll outgrow the practice of formally harmonizing with your food. One day you'll find you're just in harmony with food in general—it's your friend. Then on the odd occasion where you don't resonate with a food, you simply won't eat it. I am definitely not suggesting that you eat junk food all the time, but love what you eat or don't eat it.

You've probably outgrown the *formal* Diving In process by now. I created that method to get people back to operating the way humans were designed to operate. Once you understand and value feelings, you don't need a process to do what you're naturally designed to do: fully feel the feeling and it rises, restoring you to your Large Self power.

You will outgrow so many things in this accelerated life. If you find yourself feeling unmotivated, sluggish, stuck, or uninspired in an area of your life, even though you're generally happy, you may have outgrown something and are denying it, and that's the cause of the lower Instrument Panel reading. Life will not support you in stagnation, and will move you if you don't move, but it's more pleasant when you choose your movement consciously.

A man said he couldn't leave the abusive relationship he was in because he was loyal and had created a family—and his wife eventually divorced him. A woman was tired of her work, neglecting tasks, and slacking off—then she was fired.

It's Not Failure, It's Feedback

Okay, you've set an intention. Let it go and start walking along in your life. Everything that plays out is valuable. It's not wrong, no matter how it looks to you in any moment. It's all temporary, and it's moving.

Everything that happens is feedback, and it's showing you where your intentions are clear, or where your intentions are mixed. Things sail along smoothly where the integrity of your intention is strong. Things break down or get delayed where there's contradiction or a crack in the integrity of the intention. Use that breakdown as feedback to guide you.

Leonard Cohen's song "Anthem" says it brilliantly: "There's a crack in everything. That's how the light gets in."

Bounce off of what you don't want toward what you do want, consciously using that feeling of aversion as fuel. Use the intensity of what you don't want to propel you towards what you do want.

ACTIVITY: Harmonize With Anything

Intend vibrational alignment first: with anything—a project, upcoming meeting, a horse, a friend, or a ski slope. As it plays out, Life will give you feedback on where your intentions were clear and it worked well, or your intentions were contradicted and it didn't turn out like you wanted.

It's not failure—it's feedback.

Life Gives Feedback Along The Way

Once you set your intention, your only job is to get out of the way. Life gives you all the feedback you need to adjust and readjust your course. Pay attention to what's happening, notice how you feel, follow your inner urges, and stay in the flow. Each day Life puts the next step in front of you. You don't need to heal or fix anything, just step onto the next stepping-stone.

The process of my move to California illustrates this beautifully. Once I decided that it felt enormously right for me to move to California, my feelings ranged from ecstatic to confused, from impatient to angry. But it was all part of the valuable Instrument Panel feedback process, so those "navigational indicators" never occurred to me as wrong. I had no sense of needing to fix them, heal them, change them, or get any help with making them go away. Each feeling guided me through the necessary letting go of limits, expanding my perception, and reclaiming energy that would lead to taking the next steps.

When I sent the first email to my local community announcing the ranch was for sale, feelings arose. I felt them. The day the first offer came in, I felt my head tighten up in the beginnings of a headache. Great feedback.

One day I noticed I wasn't living as fully as I could in Austin—I had put my life on a kind of energetic hold until some future time when I was off to my new life. I didn't resist that either, but dove into that emptiness for a weekend, doing nothing, reading a novel on the front porch, wringing every drop of feeling out of it. Once that resistance softened, I dove fully back into the writing of this book, fully alive in Austin, Texas again, and the largest chunk of writing on this book was accomplished. Life's feedback is all leading you where you want to go—if you let it.

By the time I officially put my home on the market a few weeks later, life had presented me all the opportunities I needed to feel through all the feelings about letting go of my old life and beginning a new one in California.

Four months before the move, I began, step-by-step, to clear out the junk I didn't need to haul to California. Each thing I threw out moved me one step closer to an easy move. Yes, we have to take some actions, but we enjoy it more, and less action is required, when it's aligned action. Our inner genius is engaged. We're in the zone. We get more done than ten people, because we're allowing Life to assist us.

Without forcing the actions, I waited until each next step felt natural, inspired, joyful, and full of relief—with very little pushing rocks up hills. Embracing it and easing into movement in small, deliberate steps is so much easier, and as usual slow and steady action got it done faster. The attitude was, "Let it be gentle. Be nice to myself."

Consequently, within a few months, I left my thirty-eight years of life in Austin behind, and settled into Ojai with absolutely no doubts, nostalgia, regrets, or leftover feelings about moving. I moved myself one hundred percent, body, mind, spirit, and soul to California and never looked back.

So many details are taken care of for us by Grace once we set our intention to let go and get out of the way. One of my initial challenges after the move was that I left behind a whole list of ranch sitters in Austin who were always eager to enjoy a retreat there and take care of the animals while I traveled. In Ojai, we knew no one at first, and worried a bit that we'd be tied down and stuck at home. Since the beginnings of Divine Openings, worry is a mild emotion for me—nothing like the stomach knotting, knee shaking, headache inducing emotion that worry used to be. I knew this worry was contrast I'd bounce off of, and a solution would soon appear.

Sure enough, within months, Jill, a radiant being who attended a couple of retreats in Ojai and has a completely flexible schedule, volunteered to housesit for us. Then it turned out that my new assistant Susan loves to housesit. One of the former Austin ranch sitters who is a school teacher wrote, "Keep me in mind in the summer months. I'd love to come out and house-sit for you."

Life brings surprises, bonanzas, boons, and bonuses when we have strong and clear intentions and a light heart. Grace does indeed do ninety percent of everything for us, and when I'm being my Large Self, my actions produce an enormous amount of results.

Since Grace does ninety percent, our ten percent is to choose our thoughts and actions on a choice-by-choice basis. To do our best to be intentional about everything: our home, office, clothing, conversation, relationships, body, thoughts, and emotions.

If you're planning a project, a job hunt, a new business, a coffee outing, a meal, an expedition, or a romantic evening, heighten the pleasure by putting intention into it and imagining it into being, allowing plenty of flexibility for going with the flow. The setting, the sounds, scents, the dress, and the delights might be simple or they might be elaborate, but they're *intentional*.

Savor the waiting until it happens, enjoying the feeling of anticipation as much as the actual event.

Conscious intending and conscious action is not work—it *cuts down* on work. You're going to be living, thinking, doing, making choices, and taking action anyway—you might as well be doing it consciously. Adding to what I said in *Things Are Going Great In My Absence*:

To cut work to a fraction, align energy first, then take action.

* * * * * * * *

The Human Need To Be Right

One very sneaky counter-intention is the desire to be right. It hides beneath many arguments and conflicts, poses as reason and logic, and is clothed in righteousness and virtue. We know a man who threw tons of money and valuable time into writing a book that had essentially no value except to show how wrong his ex-wife and his father were. To write that book he gave up time he could have used to feel good, and make thousands of dollars of income.

It's common for the need to be right to show up as an unexpected guest in human interactions. The desire to love and honor, or create and collaborate with the other person may be the stated intention for both players—then a conflict arises, and suddenly the desire to be right rears its head. The desire to be right can temporarily overthrow the stated intention to love or collaborate.

All of us came about the need to be right honestly, so have compassion for yourself and others about it. In prehistoric times the feedback that told early man he was wrong was often injury or instant death. You did it wrong—the mastodon got you. You ate the wrong berry—you were dead.

Being wrong was deadly, and being right was so critically tied to survival that humans of course developed an incredibly strong need to be right. Your prehistoric predecessors needed to identify and choose the *right* path—life depended on it.

The mind is a wrong-seeking missile—true—but we hate it most when it finds us wrong! "I can't admit that what I've been doing all these years wasn't working! That would make me wrong!" In the grip of our pre-historic primitive brain, being wrong feels gut wrenchingly threatening, as if that mastodon is charging at us right now. As we awaken to our enlightened minds we find that getting out of sync with our Large Selves is much more painful than being wrong. It's all relative.

Of course you want to be heard and valued, and I'm not suggesting you give that up expressing what you believe in, but with clear intentions you can have it all.

ACTIVITY: Taming The Counter-Intention To Be Right

Your Larger intention is of course to support, appreciate, and connect; yet the mind can have powerful counter-intentions that contradict that.

When the desire to be right has joined the party, you might as well forget factual discussion, because when the logic is tainted with negative emotion the mind can wield it as a weapon. As always, rather than resisting your own or anyone else's resistance, recognize this strong human desire to be right, and ease up rather than pushing harder. Lean back emotionally and breathe.

If you're in the midst of a "discussion" with someone in which each of you is determined to prove yourself right, take a physical break if you can, to allow both of you to feel through your feelings. Feel the need to be right and dive into it. Soften your attitude. Refocus on your prime intentions, and recommit to your intention to connect or collaborate.

Don't argue in bed if you're lovers. Get up and go to the living room and sit facing each other. If you're co-workers, choose an appropriate setting.

The point of this powerful activity is to hear and be heard, not debate right or wrong. When you're ready to talk, intend to listen, and take time to feel and breathe while the other party speaks. Feel any tightness in your head and body from needing to be right—don't resist it, but don't give in to it either.

Take turns speaking. You can direct this informally by suggesting, "You talk first, and I'll listen without interruption for ten or fifteen minutes." Make soft eye contact and listen. People think more about what they're saying when they are looking each other in the eyes. Then, say you'd like to take your turn while the other listens without interrupting.

Begin with appreciation. "Our relationship is important to me. I respect you and want us to resolve this. I appreciate that you're so open."

Speak in terms of what you feel or think, not what someone else *did:*

> *"That part of it felt terrible,"* rather than, "You hurt my feelings."

> "This part worked, but *I felt disrespected when….*" rather than, "What you said was so disrespectful of me."

> "*I felt* good about this, but *not so good* when that happened…" rather than, "You shouldn't have said or done that horrible thing."

> "That *seems* risky to me and *I felt* left out of the decision," rather than, "You made that decision without doing enough research or consulting me."

Statements like, "YOU did this," or "YOU were wrong," take you deeper into right/wrong territory, and no matter how right you are, the other party's resistance increases. Your intention is to convey *how things felt to you or landed for you,* not to win the argument or place blame. When you talk entirely about you and *your experience* and feelings, the other person's resistance relaxes or disappears.

Say how you felt, rather than what you think about their behavior, which keeps you out of judgment. People disagree. People misinterpret and misunderstand. People get emotional and it escalates. When you lead with your Large Self and your intention is to honor the greatness in others, their Large Self steps up to meet you.

This activity soothes the primitive beast in us that needs to be right, allowing our Larger, prime intention of connection to be restored. Usually the "issues" become non-issues, requiring no further discussion. Being right isn't usually about the issues anyway—it's more about being right!

Have further discussion if necessary, but stay soft. You might come out of it still disagreeing, but honoring each other and able to go forward productively.

* * * * * * * *

Divine Timing?

Lots of us used to talk about Divine Timing. Then one day I had the epiphany that most of the time Divine Timing was another metaphysical myth we used as an excuse, to justify delays rather than claiming our own power to resist or to allow it in.

We can come up with so many comical excuses for why we're not getting what we want. "It took so long for me to get there because of Divine Timing," or "Mercury was in retrograde." Even if Mercury in retrograde was scientifically proven to be a good excuse for failure, I would still claim *my* power and give none to Mercury in *my reality.*

Nowadays I'd rather playfully say, "It took me so long to let it in because I was a stubborn donkey's ass," rather than citing Divine Timing, cosmic alignment, or any other excuse that would give my power to outside forces.

I like to say, "I created that," and get clear about my role in it as quickly as possible. If there's much of a delay, it's always me—it's not The Presence withholding what I want. The Presence creates instantly, and it can appear quickly in the physical if I'm lined up with it.

Another thing I'd say in the past was, "If we don't see something yet, it's still cooking." Then I realized that usually *it* wasn't still cooking, *I was still cooking. It* was cooked and ready the moment I wanted it, but I was not allowing it in yet. Just admitting this helps you reclaim power. When you say *it's* still cooking, or make it somehow out of your control, you forfeit power.

It doesn't take The Presence two years to deliver something, but it might take me that long to develop a skill, as with my singing. Once I set the intention, it was about two years from starting singing lessons to making my first recording of original songs. That was making pretty good time, and I was relaxed, having fun, with little pressure or resistance. I was cooking.

With my slower development in the realm of romantic relationships, The Presence could have delivered it years ago—but it took me longer to let it in.

Divine Timing *can* come into play—in this physical dimension some things *do* take a while to assemble, just as a baby takes nine months to gestate, but most of the time, it's us holding up the show. You'll learn to feel whether you're still cooking, or whether it really is Divine Timing.

Ask yourself is IT still cooking,
or is it ME that's still cooking?

I must have cooked for over a year on this book. One morning, as I tried to meditate, large pieces of it came to mind fully cooked, with no intellectual effort; so I eagerly sat down to write.

At this level of feeling and appreciation for the Instrument Panel, I feel what's coming long before it gets here. Long ago when a teacher talked about her ability to download original information like that, I was envious. If you can't yet do that you will soon. You'll feel a causeless thrill or a blast of exhilaration before you even know how the coming event could possibly occur. This is another part of that phenomenon I call *skipping to the payoff.* You get to savor that good feeling long before "it" gets here, and that good feeling *is the biggest payoff of all.*

Feeling good is a sign of something good coming.

Of course you can also feel things lining up in a way you're *not going to like* in plenty of time to shift your feelings, clear up counter-intentions, and thus realign your trajectory and change the outcome.

Intend to enjoy, surf, and appreciate pre-manifestational energy before any material evidence of it arrives. Let your feelings be as valuable to you, if not more valuable, than any material manifestation.

There's nothing to work on. Enjoy life and know that you and your awareness are expanding right now.

Your job is to feel good.

More About Timing

So if neither Divine Timing, or karma, or the planets can be blamed for slow fulfillment of an intention, what is a reasonable timetable for it to materialize? Here's the red flag: if there's any concern about timetables, you're in the way. I know you need it or you want it right now—it's just counterproductive to pulse the "it's not here" signal or fret about it.

This is where so many people get hung up. They know and feel their true Non-Physical instant manifestation power, so it can drive them crazy if it's not showing up quickly in the physical. In their distress, they nosedive and start pulsing the lack of it, and reverse or delay the materialization.

Sometimes they go back to seeking, thinking there's some magic bullet, some esoteric formula that will make it happen. It's not for lack of knowledge that it's not happening! What's worse is: when you seek you're claiming you don't have the power within, and when you say you don't have the power, the Universe has to agree with you!

Physical materialization is usually superfast for me, but not always—I've had plenty of personal experience with things taking varying amounts of time to materialize. It all depends on how clearly my broadcast tower is pulsing on that subject, which is affected by how contradicted I am. It depends on how long it takes me to live into to it, lighten up, and get out of the way.

You already know the greatest key to speeding up materialization is to *skip to the payoff*—identify the feeling you want, and start feeling it now. But if you're trying to feel better just to manipulate the manifestation process, it's inauthentic and doesn't work. Get happy simply so you can enjoy the happiness now.

Put your focus on how you want to feel rather than the material
for only one reason: because it works better.

I have lots of tangible examples of how it's worked in my life: at the beginning of Divine Openings I was on fire and unconflicted about creating Divine Openings and getting it out into the world, so it ramped up steadily and continues to. I started small because I needed that evolution. I wouldn't have been ready for a world stage at the start. I had some resistances and needed to sand off some rough edges. Experience accomplished that and the process continues.

As my consciousness expanded The Divine could speak ever more clearly through me. You see channeling comes in energy, not words, and it requires translation from pure Non-Physical impulse to physical human language. You could say I'm translating pure Non-Physical energy and intention. That evolution is still underway, and I continue to expand, let in more, and find newer and better ways to say things. You'll notice that evolution in the language of each book and course I've created. Truth expands and evolves, as do we.

Early on, a woman contacted me saying she wanted to tell her email list of a million people about

Divine Openings. I knew I was not ready to handle that yet, logistically or vibrationally, so I put her off for two months while I got ready. It was a wild and exciting time that stretched my ability to get up to speed with the energy of my Large Self and create a website that would do the mailing justice. Inner wisdom said, "don't rush it" even though my mind said "it might go away if you don't do it soon." It didn't go away; it waited for me to get ready.

Over the years I learned how to explain this nebulous thing called Divine Openings more clearly, counsel in a whole new way, get the word out so people knew I was here, create a website, learn better ways to record audios, make videos, and hone a thousand other physical-world skills. That didn't happen overnight. Sometimes I was more in the flow than others, and yes, there were speed bumps. I got frustrated. I created obstacles. I got past them. I focused on being happy during the whole journey, and still do.

Any of these steps that might have seemed difficult or slow at the time were vehicles that grew *me* as Divine Openings grew. Even if some steps could have been skipped, would I have wanted to skip them? If you could skip all the gradual unfolding of your life, and skip to the triumphant last day of your life, would you?

Why would someone play chess with another person for hours when she could simply arrange the board for the end move, eliminate the stress of competition, play chess by herself—and win every time?

Why doesn't a mountain climber just hire a helicopter to drop him off at the peak? Really? Why doesn't a marathoner just drive to the finish line and walk across it? Why don't we simply read the happily-ever-after part at the end of the novels, and watch only the ends of movies? It would save time and we'd avoid all kinds of challenges and headaches.

Each step in any life is an opportunity to experience enjoy, appreciate, expand, get feedback, learn, and grow. I don't mean learn lessons—please—this is an adventure, not an eternal school you never get to graduate from! I deliberately opted out of the lesson paradigm, by intention. I really mean enjoy, appreciate, expand, learn, and grow, not be "taught a lesson".

Before they were booked on her show, Oprah's people investigated every potential guest's business infrastructure—they knew that too large an influx of business could overwhelm an organization's ability to handle it—with disastrous results. A few people had reported that being on her show bankrupted their business when the phone rang more often than they could answer it or fulfill orders, while their regular customers were blocked by busy signals. A friend of mine was on Oprah and it did crash her website's host server for about an hour, but she recovered, and her automated site could handle the new memberships.

Babies develop in the womb over time for good reason. This is a physical world—you can't rush Life. The Presence doesn't judge and isn't worried about you if your evolution is slow, so you don't need to fret about that either. The Presence never worries at all but is so strongly vibrating love, limitless possibilities, and ecstasy that details and downsides are overridden. You cannot mess it up! You can feel it when you soften, relax, and let go, pulsing to the rhythm of your Large Self.

Romantic relationship was for a long time more challenging for me than any other area. I am independent, I have high expectations, and I'm commitment resistant. I've been divorced since 1983! I've had long-term relationships but I've never re-married.

Should The Presence wave a magic wand over me and change that? I don't think so—although honestly there were times I wished it would. I've enjoyed a gradual unfolding, celebrating the

Instrument Panel's accurate feedback at each step, lovingly and accurately showing me "Here's what you're vibrating and here's what that materializes... How does that feel? Okay, now, here's what you're vibrating and here's the product of that... How does that feel?"

My love life is fabulous and getting better by the year. The Presence is playing to my love of humor; right now, two doves are cooing and courting on the deck rail five feet from me.

Intend a love affair with the Non-Physical.

Life's contrasts guide us. It's like playing the childhood game where you're blindfolded, and the other child who can see calls out "Warmer, colder, colder... oh, boy, freezing... warmer, colder... oh, warmer, warmer, warmer, oh YES!"

The Presence is the child who can see. Her voice is your Instrument Panel. Although your Larger Self sees and knows everything, the human you plays this adventurous game, pretending to be a limited being, which adds the elements of unfolding movement in time and space and surprise.

As the time for something to materialize approaches, I can feel the "warmer, warmer!" energy heat up so tangibly that sometimes it seems impossible that it hasn't already appeared. I'll tell friends, "It's so close I can almost taste it!" Signs and omens sometimes add to the anticipation—two hawks circling overhead; walking outside into a flock of butterflies that appear from nowhere and swarm all around me. Interestingly, now I live where two hawks circling nearby at eye level is a common sight—I've even seen four. It's escalating!

When you're tapped in, you feel the Non-Physical energy first as your new creation nears physical materialization. It's often more intense than the appearance of the materialized creation, because the Non-Physical is the more potently real of the two, and the larger share of the creative process happens there. By the time it happens, you're up to speed with that energy.

The more you know and feel the Non-Physical as your prime reality, the more you are aware of your Non-Physical creations while they're still just a matrix of intention, long before they flesh out enough to show up in the physical dimension. How do you develop this capacity? Intend it and walk that talk by giving the Non-Physical more of your attention than the physical. And when the physical seems to show no evidence of what you've intended, you're so solidly anchored in the Non-Physical you won't leak power.

When you allow yourself to relax into that adventure, and let it all be feedback instead of frustration, you zoom. Even when it doesn't feel good you appreciate the valuable opportunities in it.

* * * * * * * * *

The Touch Of A Gnat's Wing

You've heard about non-attachment, but please clear your mind of any pre-existing definitions of non-attachment, and hear this fresh. When I use the word "non-attachment" I do not mean letting go of attachment to all earthly things. I don't believe in that—I think it's misguided.

Believe what you choose to—my view is that we came to a physical world to enjoy it—not to ignore it, resist it, get out of it, or sacrifice it so we can get to Heaven. Wanting more is as natural and essential as breathing, and it drives the evolution of all species, and indeed of the entire Universe.

What I mean by non-attachment is staying light and calm about something we want so that we're not white-knuckle gripping it, which creates resistance and slows down its arrival. Being too attached is getting in the way. The easiest way to speed up the arrival of what you want is to take as light and easy an attitude about it as you can muster. It can be challenging until it becomes your habit, but let's face it—the alternative (resistance) is ten times more challenging.

The lighter the intention, the faster the creation can appear. While writing my Level Two Online Retreat Course, I was looking for a way to help people viscerally *feel* just how lightly to intend, when these words came to me, "Make your intention as light as the touch of a gnat's wing." I also put those words in my song "Heaven" in the *Watch Where You Point That Thing* music collection that inspired the title of this book.

Intend as lightly as the touch of a gnat's wing. It helps you to intend and then let it go, knowing it's coming, or that something that will fulfill your heart's desires even better will appear. When you let go, the forces of the Universe can go to work on your behalf, unencumbered by your resistance.

A practical definition for resistance
in this context is "tension."

Granted, it's a measure of your mastery to see how unattached you can be when you want or need something enormously and you need it soon. For many of you, to materialize things like someone giving you a blue shirt in the style you imagined, or have a friend call just when you were thinking about them, or have small checks arrive unexpectedly is easy, but when it comes to materializing the big things like love, healing from a serious illness, or getting out of debt, you might tense up and add resistance.

It's easier with small creations only because of *how you feel about them*: the stakes are low, you aren't tense or stressed about it, and so are not too attached. You are relaxed. You don't *doubt* those small miracles are possible for you. With bigger desires, you might doubt that they are possible, and that negative counter-intention gets in the way. The bigger your intention, the more you need to let it go. Bigger things can arrive just as magically and easily as the small things.

When you visualize, intend, or imagine—do it lightly—as if for pleasure. Rest in it, fantasize about it lightly, feel it as if it's already yours, and quickly let it go.

People sometimes say, "I want it in a bad way."
It works better to want it in a good way!

There's no need to *hold* the intention, work at it, or try to sustain it. Working too hard is counterproductive, because it adds tension, and thus resistance, to the materialization process, and demonstrates doubt that it can come that easily. More than 99% of the work of creation is done with your intention. Universal Intelligence instantly hears what you want. Then your job is to let The All That Is bring everything together in perfect synchronicity and perfect timing. It can best do that without you in the way.

Another way to say it is, "Focus without force."

Make your intentions as light as the touch of a gnat's wing.

You're Not Separate From It

"Ask, knowing it is given" is ancient wisdom, but being able to conjure up the physical feeling and the knowing that *it is given* has been the great challenge throughout the ages. You look around and it's not here. You feel your feelings, and they feel like it's not here either.

The Bible tells us to have faith—that's a tough one, too. As you know, I never ask you to have faith, because you don't need faith—evidence is much better, and you can generate some feeling evidence almost immediately, long before you get the physical evidence. Feelings *are* the prime manifestation you wanted.

Here are some ways to viscerally feel the reality of what you want—and to close the gap between what you want and its arrival.

Everything in the Universe is One. No one and nothing is actually separate from you. You are everyone and everyone is you. You and your worst enemy are one, no matter how it looks from your human perspective.

You are one with the farthest reaches of this and all Universes. The mind, that wrong seeking missile and separation machine, tells you everything is separate from you, but there is no such separation.

Space, time, and limiting boundaries are illusions we agree to live by when we come here, but we don't have to believe in them so slavishly. At any moment you can choose to experience yourself as part of a holographic Universe—everything is in you—nothing is actually separate from you.

If a loved one has left her body, she is not removed from you. Your beloved pet or your grandmother may appear to be deceased, but in the Oneness they are more alive than you, and right here with you, completely aware of you. If someone dear to you lets go of his physical body, it can actually be the most incredible gift he's ever given you if you let it in. In *Things Are Going Great In My Absence* I suggested cultivating a close, personal, relatable concept of The Presence, and it can get even easier once this human person you felt so close to on Earth becomes wholly Non-Physical—it can be a bridge to the Non-Physical realm for you. Tune in to the high frequencies where they are, and you can feel or even talk with them. Focus on them, and your intention alone brings the connection.

While I deliberately focus on the Non-Physical and give scant attention to material manifestation, get ready for this power-packed sentence: you and whatever *physical* person, thing, or experience you want *are already one*. Recognize that, vibrate that reality, feel it in the Non-Physical, and you will experience it.

For some of you who have had that "big opening" or have practiced softening, this short, simple section is phenomenally powerful. Stop now and recognize your oneness with what you want.

Claim your oneness with what you want.
You are not separate from it.

* * * * * * * *

Your Reservoir

You know, I always say things in different ways and at different levels. If you're not quite ready to let in the truth that you are already one with what you want, a great way to get your mind out of the way when it's lackfully lamenting, "It's not here yet," is to feel into your Reservoir. In the Non-Physical there actually exists a giant energetic reservoir where everything you've ever wanted is held for you until you let it in. Lower vibrations on the Instrument Panel keep the floodgates partly closed, although the goodness of Life always insures there is some flow to you. You already know your job is not to work on yourself or muscle the floodgates open, but to shift those feelings, soften, and let it in.

Of course, it's not a physical lake at all, but the image of a giant lake does help the human mind grasp it. You might see it as something other than a lake. It's your reservoir so it can take on any form you like.

This is not merely a metaphor. It is real in the Non-Physical, and once something's in your reservoir it's one vibrational shift away from popping into the physical. As the Non-Physical becomes more and more real to you, you'll feel the reality of this reservoir and everything in it.

People want everything they want because they think it will make them feel better—that it's the key to their happiness. Skip to the payoff. Feel it in your reservoir right now. Get happy now.

It's already created. It's already yours.
It's in the reservoir.

ACTIVITY: Visit Your Reservoir Meditation (audio in Level Two Online)

As you think of people, circumstances, or pure feelings you desire to bring into your life, take a little trip, and visit your reservoir. Notice all the things in it. Maybe your ideal lover is paddling a kayak on the reservoir. Maybe your new job is there. Over there you see your next level of joy and freedom, your fun new friends, some exotic travel, and your deeper Oneness with The Presence that gives you total peace in life. Your happy old age is there, along with your increased wisdom and creativity.

There's a party going on at this reservoir, and everyone is waiting for you to arrive and feel these feelings waiting for you. It's your party.

Dive into the reservoir for a refreshing swim in the good feelings waiting there for you. Or fly around it, visiting aspects of this creation of yours. Soothe yourself by saying and feeling, "It's already created. It's already mine. It's all right here." This is not just an affirmation—it is true in the Non-Physical. Saying it just helps you line up with the truth.

Relax and savor the good feelings!

Once you feel it, it's drawing nearer, so soothe yourself to keep that good feeling good. And don't get stuck on how you think it should be or look. Let The Presence fill all that in.

The house we moved into in Ojai had been severely neglected, and we wanted to get it livable quickly so we could get back to work. For example, the house had cement floors and exposed tack strips because the previous owners had ripped out the carpet, then couldn't afford to replace it. There were so many essential things to be done at once that when, in a single week, we got new carpet, new tile, a new water heater, new electrical plugs, new paint, new barn, the roof fixed, and scores of other things spruced up, there wasn't that delicious opportunity to appreciate each new thing one by one. But now, I want to draw out my appreciation.

Right now I'm delaying hooking up the hot tub I brought here from Texas ten months ago. We've done so many things to make this house wonderful, and I prefer to savor and enjoy each of those things fully, one by one, rather than rushing on to the next thing. Each new flowering plant, each new added convenience in the barn, each new dab of paint is a distinct pleasure.

Savoring the waiting for the hot tub is fun, and when it's hot and steaming on some chilly evening this winter, I'll enjoy it all the more for not having had it for a while. I'm happy now. It can wait.

Savor the waiting as you would a visit from your lover.

The mind might say we need all our desires fulfilled right now, but it's surprising how much more satisfying it is to enjoy the coming of each experience, each thing, each person, each expansion, each moment, step by step, for the whole journey, taking time to savor each new development.

There is no shame in not letting everything come to you instantly. We all expand and evolve over time, and we let it in when we're ready, but it makes you feel better to remind yourself that it's not being withheld from you—it's in your reservoir.

So many people write me to say that when they got themselves feeling better, things began to shift. Paradoxically, once they felt that good, they often didn't care so much about all the "stuff" they once thought was the key to their happiness. Once they got happy the importance of all that faded, then what they wanted started showing up anyway.

While progress might have seemed slow at the time, when they looked back after a year, they barely recognized their lives. If reading about other people's physical evidence helps you raise your vibration, read some of the thousands of notes at DivineOpenings.com/testimonials.

Summary: Savor the waiting and enjoy the time between now and the arrival of your creation. Remind yourself it's already yours. It's in your reservoir, so enjoy the good feeling now. That good feeling forms a matrix that attracts good things.

* * * * * * * *

Do I Need To Visualize?

There's no need to visualize to create something—it's already yours! Visualize for the same reason you put the kids in front of an entertaining video so you can get some work done. The Presence needs you relaxed and not fretting so your creation can be cooked up without you in the way. Things go great in your absence. Visualize to keep *yourself* happy and entertained. Daydream simply to *feel* the good vibration of having it—*now*.

When you're not thinking about what you've intended, at least you're not contradicting it, doubting, or vibrating counter-intentions. It's better to go take a nap than get in the way. Meditating to "work on it" also gets you in the way—what you want is in your reservoir—meditate to enjoy the feeling of having it. The moment you wanted it, The Presence created it, and said, "Here—it's yours. You were never separate from it, but if you can't let it in yet, I'll hold it in the reservoir till you can." You can let go and relax now.

Visualizing for any reason except for pleasure is like nagging—The Presence has a perfect memory, heard your desire the first time, and has already created it in the Non-Physical and put it in your reservoir. Open the floodgates and let it into your life.

If daydreaming and visualizing in a light, easy way keeps your mind productively occupied, relaxes your body, and soothes your soul, do it. If it leads to persistent tension, thoughts of not having it, or working at it, stop. Don't resist your resistance. If you're daydreaming along nicely, and counter-intentions or doubts come up, dive into the feeling until it rises. Or stop and think about something else to get out of the way.

Visualize purely for pleasure.

Get creative if the reservoir image doesn't resonate with you. Visualize and daydream of your bank vault, hidden cave, or open a time capsule and read a newspaper article proving your creation has already happened in the future. Play with it. Use your imagination. Rave about how it felt.

Vision Boards

Making a vision board is not a new idea, but this approach is: Your desires were granted to you the minute you intended them, you're never separate from what you want, so don't make a vision board to create anything—the creation's already done. The vision board just helps you *skip to the payoff* and summon the new feeling that creates the new matrix. It reminds you of your oneness with your desire and helps you feel it.

Get a sheet of foam core or poster board. Paste pictures on the board to represent the *feelings and life experiences* you want to create rather than the physical things. You can add feeling words: ease, joy, love, accomplishment, self-esteem, adventure, vitality, energy, flow, friendship, support, appreciation, freedom, comfort, etc.

You can use pictures of physical things you want, or words such as home, savings, relationship, travel, but leaving it general and open-ended allows for better outcomes. If you don't get stuck on visiting some specific country or marrying some specific person, The Presence can bring something even better. For years, a teenage girl dreamed of and visualized marrying a certain mega-famous movie star. She put his picture on her vision board, and years later she did get him, but he's not quite what she thought—he's gay but not willing to be who he is, and needed a wife to be his "beard."

Hang your vision board where you can see it and enjoy the unfolding of your desires. Then, make a new board with fresh desires. I love checking off each item after a year has passed.

You, Inc.

If you'd like to create a new job or career, first consider that studies show people take for granted or undervalue their natural gifts, erroneously believing that if it's easy for them it must not be valuable, and that if it required more struggle it would be more valuable. Nothing could be further from the truth. Follow what is natural, easy, and joyful for you. Observing from Large Self Perspective, your unique and even odd combination of talents, experiences, interests, and knowledge are a perfect fit for something. Ask your friends and employers to list your gifts—they'll mention things you didn't even realize have value.

Make a "marketing package" about you. Design it like a report or product booklet, and you're the product. Create sections highlighting each of your skills, gifts, and experiences, and illustrate it colorfully with pictures of you and your work, conveying how you want your next phase to feel. Put it in a beautiful binder, put Your Name, Inc. on the cover and adore it until you *sell yourself on yourself*. It is The Presence expressing as you.

When I first did this, I played with it until I was sold on me. I hired a professional photographer to take the pictures, proposed exactly what I'd do to serve the specific needs of a company I wanted to work with, and the manager created an entirely new position to fit my diverse set of talents.

Visions boards and You, Inc., packages help you skip to the payoff, and ease into the new vibration you desire rather than pushing rocks up hills.

ACTIVITY: Vision Board and You, Inc. Party - These activities are fun to do with friends. You can point out each other's talents. Don't just read about this—experience it!

* * * * * * * *

Don't Wait, Generate

You are a veritable generator of feelings, blood chemicals, energy matrices, vortexes, and vibrations. If you could only hear your "generator" humming away in response to your own thoughts, feelings, and intentions, you'd be amazed. Actually, some of you already *can* hear and feel it humming away—you feel the chemicals squirting into your bloodstream as you think this thought or that.

Whatever you intend happens more quickly when you generate the energies, feelings, and thoughts you want rather than hoping they show up.

Being "at the effect of" the people and circumstances around us is a hard way to live. You know how that goes: happy if the partner is loving—miserable if not; happy if the boss approves—stressed if not; secure if there's extra money in the bank—anxious if not; prosperous if the economy is good—struggling if not. Those outer stimuli are just things to bounce off of as you correct your course.

Most people will agree with you if you say, "The way it's going out there determines my emotions," or "I will feel secure when I have a job." But you know you don't ever have to wait for the physical pieces to fall into your lap to be happy. You can generate happiness from nothing, anytime. You can *skip to the payoff* and be happy now, plus speed up your desired materialization.

One day I noticed that the word "en-joy" literally means *put the joy into*—not wait for it to happen, or hope it will happen. Believing joy is something that happens to you leaves you powerless and dependent. *Generate* feelings and states of being instead of passively waiting for them.

When you en-joy it you put the joy into your experience.

Things Are Going Great In My Absence and Level One Online ask you to practice raving—you talk up what you appreciate until you're literally buzzing with that high vibration. You don't just mouth the words intellectually; you juice them up with passion and power. You feel your vibration rise, long before a single thing changes in your outer world. You *skip to the payoff*, feel happier first, and then watch new things appear in your life to match your newly generated matrix.

Raving is a proactive choice, as opposed to waiting for outer evidence or something to make you happy. Some reserved people resist raving, feeling it's inauthentic, undignified, or even bragging; but not choosing to generate makes us mere passive reactors to or even victims of whatever happens to be going on out there.

Generating works, because, yes, you get more of what you focus on and what you dramatize and pump up. Point your mind in productive directions and you create the evidence and see the results.

In his humorous and insightful book, *The Guinea Pig Diaries: My Life As An Experiment,* author A.J. Jacobs actually *becomes* more refined and gallant as he acts out George Washington's *Rules of Civility* in daily life. When he bows as he meets people, he feels more respectful; when he writes careful, formal letters to resolve conflicts he feels more rational; by reining in anger he feels wiser. Exercising when you're tired makes you feel more energetic, and raving makes you feel optimistic. Don't wait for the feeling to find you—actively *generate it.*

Don't merely "ask, knowing it is given"—instead, "intend, knowing you are the creator of it." Don't wait for evidence, feel it here, now.

If you want to truly feel and know your Large, Unlimited, Non-Physical Self, intend it—just choose it rather than striving for it. Don't ask if you're worthy—claim it. It is that simple, and the more you choose expansion and joy, the more that becomes your reality.

Don't passively wait—generate.

* * * * * * * *

A Physical Rave

Let's take raving one giant step farther. Moving your body adds power. There's a physiology that accompanies every emotion. Try this right now. Hunch your shoulders and droop. Let your face go slack and half-close your eyes. This is the physiology of fatigue, discouragement, or depression. In this posture, you're not generating energy.

Now, raise your hands to the ceiling and wave them around. Smile broadly, open your eyes wide, and move your head side to side. You're generating energy now. It pumps up your raving because it's physically congruent with raving. Your face and body usually display your vibration, although it is entirely possible to be blissed out and look blasé.

Our thoughts, feelings, blood chemistry, ways of moving our bodies, and our emotions are far more habitual than we realize. By freeing the body of rigid habitual ways of moving, we also free ourselves from habitually limiting ways of thinking, feeling, and being in life.

We form default vibrational, emotional,
mental, and movement habits.

When you get stuck in an unproductive thought or feeling and want to shake it off, or if you just want to *generate* a higher high, get up and move rather than trying to think your way there. The chemistry of your entire body changes as your body and blood flow more freely.

Yes, intention is powerful, but it's even more powerful when you act consistently with that intention, telling your entire system you really mean business. For example, you can intend to exercise, and talk excitedly about exercising, but your muscles start increasing in size only after you pick up the weights and start lifting. You can intend to write a book, and talk passionately about writing your book, but when you put pen to paper or begin to type, your whole being knows you mean it.

We say lots of things. Do them.

I've practiced non-habitual movement for years, and its power is demonstrated most dramatically in the Five Day Silent Retreats. People in very low vibrations, especially numb, fat-shielded, or depressed people who usually take longer to feel their feelings, find that non-habitual movement loosens them up faster. Of course, the field of resonance is a powerful factor, but movement helps them Dive In, let go, and fly higher then and afterward. We simply don't realize how strongly emotion is tied to physiology.

My music CD, *Watch Where You Point That Thing* comes with access to a web video showing you how to do non-habitual movement. It's available on our website at DivineOpenings.com/spiritual-enlightenment-music. I'll share how to do non-habitual movement here, but it's easier when you can see it and follow along. That music is a perfect complement to this book.

ACTIVITY: Non-Habitual Movement

How to do non-habitual movement:

1. Put on music that inspires you to move.
2. Move through the emotions, beginning with any lower emotions you're experiencing, and act your way up to feelings you want to feel.
3. Begin with very subtle slow warm-up movements, bending and stretching, but don't do your same old habitual movements. Do only movements you've never done before.
4. After the warm-up, move your body in the stupidest, most ridiculous-looking ways you can possibly dream up. Feel through any resistance to doing this!
5. Keep catching yourself doing habitual movements, and do something outrageously new every fifteen seconds or so. Act like an animal, crawl on the floor, move backwards, flail and flap, act like a squid. Move each joint in a way that opens up new sensations and feelings.
6. At some point, act out being your Unlimited Non-Physical Self.
7. At the end, lie down and let go. Feel the contrast of sound and silence, movement and stillness, and the new vibrations you generated.

Get up and do it right now. If you resist doing it, recognize the counter-intention to stay in old habits and comfort zones. If the counter-intention is stronger than the intention for expansion, the counter-intention wins. Will you let that happen or get proactive?

Set the intention to generate feelings of your own choice rather than waiting for feelings to happen to you. It's much more fun than letting circumstances be the cause and you simply reacting to them.

I've been sitting and writing too much lately, and right now my body is telling me to get up and move. I am committed to walking my talk, because mere talk is cheap. If I didn't do these things myself, you'd feel the lack of integrity, and my power of intention would suffer. Can't have that! Plus, resisting hurts, and relief feels really good.

I'll be back in a while.

When you're the generator, you're at cause,
and Life responds to you.

* * * * * * * *

You're Either A Sponge Or A Leader

Let's further clarify how you either generate your own vibration or let it be determined for you. After a recent session with me, a woman had a huge breakthrough in her happiness and health when she understood that she'd been letting the world and those around her set her vibratory level. She was looking for approval, trying to be compassionate, and like many women, she felt it was her job to feel *their* feelings and fix them.

She was a "sponge" for what everybody else was thinking, feeling, and radiating rather than a Leader deliberately generating the vibration of her own choice. "I thought that's what love was!" she declared.

You're either a Sponge, or a Leader. You can't be both. One client became a leader, and her entire family is transforming—even her macho dad calls on her now for uplifting and soothing, although he wouldn't admit it—he's just calling to "chat." In her childhood and early adulthood she had been a Sponge by default. Now she knows better, and chooses to be a vibrational Leader.

The country gets more prosperous when the news says "the economy" is booming, and people get poorer when the news says the economy is bad. Why is that? It's because Sponges can only prosper if there's prosperity vibration out there to sponge up. They don't generate. They follow the herd instead of leading.

When everyone hears how bad the economy is, the news nose-dives vibration for many across the country, businesses go bust, and people can't find jobs. They're sponging. There is the same amount of money and goods as ever. There is no such thing as "the economy"—it's an illusion people can buy into, or not. We each create our own economy. People who innocently sponge up low vibration and bad news are not creating their own reality—they're letting the government, media, or peers lead them and tell them what their reality is. Most people read this, set their intention, and stop sponging, but if you have difficulty there is an excellent article to help you at DivineOpenings.com. Search Free Articles.

As each new roomful of blissed out people leave the Five-Day Silent Retreat, I remind them that they have been in my field of resonance twelve hours a day for five days—plus the preparatory period when they, by intention, allow themselves to be gradually ramped up for the retreat. I remind them that I've been holding a very high vibration, which they easily sponged up and were supported by. I've been the Leader, navigator, and driver. But to maintain and expand their bliss they must learn to drive themselves. If they venture out into the world as a Sponge, or go back to seeking and letting other people drive for them, they abdicate power and go backwards.

You as The Presence are the rightful Leader in your own life. If I get the guidance to do so, I'll let in help, but only from someone who points me back to my own powerful Inner Being. Build your inner power rather than relying on outside crutches, people, seeking, and modalities.

The Presence will never say, "Okay, you're enlightened and blissed out now, and I will never let you leave this vibration again." No, you have Free Will, and that is a good thing. You can surf it all, appreciating all feelings as good and valuable, navigating powerfully along your way, or you can turn the steering wheel over to other people, and go back to that old reality.

It's always going to be a choice. Be your own Leader.

You're either a Sponge or a Leader.

ACTIVITY: Increase Your Radiance

This meditative activity is useful for daily recharging, prevention from sponging up others' vibrations, letting go of anything you did sponge up, generating power, physical energy, health, mental clarity, relief, or to give yourself a treat instead of a fix.

Close your eyes and simply intend to amp up your pinging, pulsing, beaming, radiating core. When you focus on your own Large Self's resonance, it dominates so powerfully there's no room for any other vibration in your entire energy field. You don't have to see it, *just intend and feel it.*

It might feel overwhelming initially, so take it easy at first. That is how your Large Self beams *all the time,* and this literally takes you physically into your expanded Large Self State. It's a great morning meditation—it only takes a few seconds, but you could enjoy it longer.

* * * * * * * *

Right Here Right Now

Your power is always right here and right now. You haven't lost anything unrecoverable. There is no history that can't be rewritten or discarded, no karma to resolve. There is no truly fatal mistake, since there is no death and no ending to your eternal adventure.

There is no lost ancient knowledge you must find. The current new energies are more powerful than any ancient esoteric secrets or texts you might dig up, and tomorrow's new energies will be more powerful than today's, because we'll be ready for them. We expand our pipes gradually, and all we've lived before is available to us right now in this life. Knowing that your power is in the now frees you up to develop your power of intention because you aren't constantly thinking there's something else somewhere that you need.

Journeys to pyramids, vortices, and sacred sites don't interest me. Why not bring that energy and magic to the place where you are? Your vortex of power is right where you sit if you're clear and allow it. People talk about magic dates, numbers, and power spots. If you give your power to that, you'll always be looking for it "out there" or waiting for the next magical numerological date. The magic day is today.

Mercury in retrograde has never made one ounce of difference in any way for me because I give it absolutely zero power. If someone points those dates out as a potential problem, I just ignore it. It holds *them* back because they've given it power. Their cell phones may not work and their projects may stall, but mine work just fine.

People often desperately seek an outer excuse that explains what's happening to them. The problem is that perspective gives power away to some external cause rather than claiming our own power and authorship. I'd rather say, "I created it," and keep my power than abdicate power to some outer influence. Giving away power in any way *decimates your power of intention.* Giving away power says, "I'm not creating it—I'm powerless," and The Presence must agree with you.

Your power is now.
The magic date is today.
The power is within you.
The power spot?
You're sitting on it.

You have access to everything in the Universe if you really need it: past, present, future, other dimensional, all of it. You don't have to work on your past lives—any past life vibrations you're still vibrating are reflected in your current circumstances for you to feel. You don't need to dig through the past—just feel through what's in front of you right here, right now.

All the talents and gifts you came in with are accessible to you, right here, right now. You don't have to go to Egypt to find them. Just feel your Instrument Panel, start doing what calls to you step by step, and let it blossom. Intend to unfold, and let it happen. Get out of your comfort zone and try new things. Let go of resistances and fears and get out of the way.

Get solidly planted in the now, and you're freed up to explore the Universe. Stop resisting being *right here, right now,* and, paradoxically, you can go anywhere.

Before I introduce alternate realities in our Level Three Online Retreat, Jumping The Matrix, people must take the prerequisite Levels One and Two because you need to be very stable to take Jumping The Matrix. Many people who didn't believe me at first have verified this, then backed out of it till they were ready.

You see, you think you want to mess with your reality, but if you're not stable and centered squarely in your power, it can be quite disorienting when your reality wobbles and reveals itself to be less than solid. Whether you like it or not, you rely on its predictability more than you think. After familiar aspects of their less expanded identity have dissolved, many people say to me, "I don't even know who I am now that everything I used to base my identity on is gone."

In Jumping The Matrix Online, we operate under the assumption that all time, space, and other dimensions are here and now—all of it explosively diverse and infinitely creative aspects of the One. We bring selected parts of those alternate realities *into the now.* In those powerful and profound processes, you visit one of the infinite number of alternate You's who made different choices than you did, and therefore now has a different and in some ways better life than the You you're living as in this dimension. You see, we make decisions at crucial pivot points in our lives, and each of those pivot points alters the trajectory of our lives. Alternate You's made different decisions, and their lives are accordingly different.

Not All There

You've heard people use the expression, "He's not all there," when they mean someone is a little crazy or absent-minded. Here I'll use this term for someone who's not completely in his body.

Our power of intention increases when we are fully grounded in the body, on this planet, engaged in life, feeling good about it. The spiritual bypass attempts to avoid feeling the body and emotions, and diminishes your power of intention. Bring Heaven to Earth rather than trying to ascend out of here. Stop resisting being here, and be here one hundred percent.

The story tempts us to focus on how wrong the feeling is, and how wrong the situation is that gave us the feeling. *Things Are Going Great In My Absence* walked us through how best to deal with feelings, but we're human. Some of us resist in clever ways. No problem! Life continues to put us in situations that invite us to master feelings until we do it. Stay with it and relax.

If you're not all here, your power of intention is also not all here. Spiritual people who have difficulty coping with the world, money, relationships, sex, and other physical aspects of life are often "not all here."

To claim all of your power, you must be all *here.*

Getting into your body and being right-here-right-now is a vital part of mastering your power of intention. Appreciate and embrace every experience, even the ones you don't like. Stay out of the details of the story and go to a softer, more general feeling-focus to build your new matrix. Say things to yourself like, "It gets better all the time. I'm expanding day by day. Soften into this."

Embrace "what is" in every moment—make it right. Notice that "what is" is temporary. If you forget it's temporary and get too focused on any current unwanted reality, it gets recreated over and over. I certainly understand the challenge of that. I, too, experience moments when the reality of something unwanted claims way too much of my attention. And yet I've seen seemingly impossible things shift overnight when I take my attention off the problem and point it at even a vague general possibility of relief.

You can now begin to shift your reality just by setting the intention.

All you need is right here, right now.

ACTIVITY: Grounding Yourself Here And Now

There's an audio that guides you through this activity in the Self-Paced Level Two Online Retreat.

This activity has several parts. Go slowly, sensing deeply. If you read this and rush on without experiencing it physically, you'll miss the visceral experience that makes it real and powerful, and brings it down to Earth. Anytime you try to accomplish evolution in your head without grounding it in physical experience—it just doesn't work as well. Thinking is made reality by experience.

1. Focus on your physical body: Put your attention in your left hand. Lovingly stroke your right forearm with your left hand. Really experience what your left hand is feeling, with all of your senses. Note how the left hand feels, and how it picks up the temperature, texture, shape, color, and size of your right forearm. Notice any other information your left hand picks up about your right arm. Feel it and let your mind go blank.

2. Focus on pleasure rather than thoughts about what you're doing. Notice how easy or challenging this is, and be with that feeling. Make this a pleasurable activity. Feel the pleasure completely. Notice how worthy you feel to receive pleasure, or how distracted you get, and be with that feeling.

3. Now put your attention on your right forearm and feel it. Notice that your right forearm has its own set of experiences and sensations, independent of your left hand.

4. Now, move your arm slowly in the air and feel the air around your arm. What do you notice about the air? Temperature? Movement? Scents? Other sensations?

5. Listen to the sounds that surround you. In this sensitized state you notice things you hadn't before.

6. Smell the scents around you. Smell some part of your own body. Sniff your dog or cat. Inhale the scent of a candle or soap.

So now you're here, in your body. I joke that spiritual people are often unconsciously fleeing physical experience, scheming to get out of here, or aspiring to get "somewhere else." Some want out-of-body experiences or to go to other dimensions. You can visit other dimensions, but until you get happy and grounded in this one, it won't help you, and you won't be any happier or more successful in this life. In fact, when people go out of their body or off into wild spiritual experiences to escape, it makes them even unhappier when they have to return to their body.

Some want to avoid old vibrations and feelings in their bodies, which unbeknownst to them, puts a ceiling on their enlightenment. They may have had good reason to want to get out of their body, and I have compassion for that, but getting happy in your body is essential.

Divine Openings is an "in-body experience". You decided to come to this beautiful planet, so intend to get yourself *all here*, get happy and masterfully here, and enjoy it! Land on Earth!

Divine Openings is an in-body experience.

* * * * * * * *

Intend Freedom From The Past

You may indeed have reclaimed all of your power from the past. But most of us leak away small amounts of power regularly, without noticing it. It's subtle and gradual, and justified with good intentions, so it's helpful to intend to keep yourself freed up. At every Five Day Retreat—about four times a year—I notice if I've leaked any power, and if so, I bring it back home. Nobody took it from me—I gave it away and I can take it back.

Perhaps you reclaimed some before but now you're finally ready to reclaim more. Are you lamenting any past circumstance? Holding a grudge? Giving away your happiness to someone who hurt you or let you down? Mad at yourself? *Things Are Going Great In My Absence* gets most people past this, but if the resistance to feeling the feeling and dropping the story has been high, or if the allure of "being right about how wrong it was" has tempted you, you can get all your power back.

People who have had trauma in their past sometimes try to escape those feelings by being only partially in their body. Get in your body and reclaim your power. Even if after reading *Things Are Going Great In My Absence* you still find it challenging to appreciate all emotions, go back again and experience it more deeply.

You may choose to take the appropriate online First Aid Retreat or Level One online course. The recordings of my voice in those courses closely approximate live interaction with me, which is fortunate because I rarely give individual sessions anymore. The quality of your life depends on getting all your power back from past events, past traumas, people who hurt you, or whom you hurt. There is just no way to claim your full power of intention with part of your power tied up in the past. You need it here and now.

If your heart is still closed off to key people from your past, especially family, you simply must get your love pipes open and flowing. Someone may have hurt you in the past, but it you don't get free of it, *you're the one who's hurting you now.* It's astounding how much your power of intention increases when your love pipes are open. It makes sense when you feel it: open equals flow, closed even a little equals less flow. Your Large Self loves unconditionally and doesn't judge, so to judge or withhold love takes you out of alignment with your Large Self.

The most important thing of all is that your heart is open to *you.* If you're holding judgments, blame, or unworthiness, set the intention right now to let that go. You're disagreeing with The Presence.

If someone hurt you in the past and you're still vibrating that,
now it's you who is hurting you.

ACTIVITY: Intend To Reclaim Power Tied Up In Past

Stop right now and intend:

- I intend all power I have tied up in past hurts and disappointments to return to me right now. In order to get all my power back, I am willing to stop making anyone wrong and flow my love to them regardless of what they feel. I don't have to know how—I intend it.
- I intend that all power I've tied up in guilt for mistakes or for hurting others is returned to me right now. I declare that history no longer holds any of my power and I call that power back to me. I don't have to know how—I intend it.
- I intend that all power tied up in anything less than love for others is returned to me right now. I don't have to know how—I intend it.
- I intend that all power tied up in my genetic heritage be returned to me right now. I don't have to know how—I intend it.

You've intended. Now take the ride.

* * * * * * * *

Reclaim A Hundred Percent Of Your Power

Now you've set intentions, softened ties to the past or eliminated them, and committed to being right here. I find it more effective to approach one subject in several different ways—one person will hear me best when I say it one way, and another will hear it best another way.

Imagine that someone has a hundred total watts of power to use to live her life. She's a hundred-watt bulb. But is she shining at a hundred watts? Or does her power supply have a dimmer on it, dulling her radiance and her pulse?

If she still has some lower vibration humming inside her about a past relationship that didn't go well, maybe that's tying up ten watts of her power. Then there's resentment about the unfairness of not getting a promotion at work. That ties up fifteen watts of her power. Then there's fear about her future career prospects because she's getting older. That's using twenty-five watts of her power. Worry about her health is using another ten watts.

She adds it all up to find that sixty percent of her total energy is tied up, and realizes she could use that energy more productively. Forty percent of her power is humming along at a higher vibration, available for her to use, and that's actually pretty darn good—but that sixty percent that's tied up makes her tired, less powerful, and less bright and gifted than she actually is.

She has to work longer and harder to make up for not having all of her energy available. It's tough trying to overcome your own vibration—it's like flying into a headwind of your own making. It's tough trying to push rocks up hills. Everything is much easier when you have all your energy free to use as you choose.

And she's not living completely in the now. All of that sixty percent is tied up either in the past or the future. In the past, we have no power—that's all history. Our power to intend for the future is right now.

The point is not to make an accurate mathematical calculation. It's to help you be aware if any of your power is tied up, and how much of it is available to you. Once you get that insight, you can forget the numbers.

To use a computer analogy, you could say running all those extra programs saps her energy and slows down her hard drive. Have you ever had to close programs on your computer to free up power for the task at hand? This person's power of intention would be much more potent if she freed up that other sixty percent of her power.

Don't try to fix anything. It's going to start improving the moment you become conscious of it and the light of awareness shines on it. Once you get it, you begin to shift, and Life and Grace will help you.

A woman was talking with me about money problems in a course, but quickly I felt it wasn't about money—it was about her energy, power, and clarity. I could hear and feel she was operating at low wattage, so I asked her how much of her wattage was tied up. We estimated, added it up, and it was seventy percent!

She'd been imploding her anger and resentment, not letting herself feel what she felt and want what she wanted. All her years of hard work with little reward had left her complacent and resigned. She was stuck in a comfort zone and didn't have the energy to jump out of it. She'd been taking care of others first, to the point where she was drained but didn't notice it happening. It was a huge blind spot.

She reclaimed that power by pure intention. I asked her to feel into her future and experience how she would feel when she was shining at one hundred watts. "How will it feel when someone tells you their whole life got better after spending a few days with you, after you've done nothing but be yourself, beaming at a hundred watts?"

We didn't "do" anything to fix it. After the Divine Opening, her own Divine Intelligence, which she was getting more tapped into all the time and had more access to once she reclaimed her wattage, made all the adjustments, and she is now ecstatically happy. Her marriage improved immensely, and her zest for life skyrocketed. She has her power back, free to use as she chooses.

Your attention and intention are powerful instruments, and with Divine Openings, once you *see* something through your Divine Eyes, that Divinely Intelligent system you've tapped into begins to make adjustments to align you more completely with your Divine Self, your Larger Self.

Look at the Instrument Panel in *Things Are Going Great In My Absence* if you don't know it by heart by now. Scribble numbers by all the feelings as you estimate the amount of power tied up there, and add it all up. Don't worry. Power in higher vibrations is much more potent than power in lower vibrations. This isn't to scare you—it's to help you be aware of and reclaim your power so that your intentions have one hundred percent of your power behind them.

Write the answers to the following questions right here in the book. You'll enjoy coming back one day soon to find you're much more powerful.

ACTIVITY: Estimate Percentages:

How much of your power, energy, thoughts, and feelings are tied up in lower vibrations—or with regrets, losses, anger, guilt, or hurts from your past? Feel those feelings and don't make them wrong, but drop the story. You're going to get your power back!

How much of your power is tied up with people in the past?

How much of your power is tied up in concern about the future?

How much of your power is tied up in thoughts about what you don't have, or can't do right now?

How much is tied up in resistance to what you don't want to do, or are afraid to do?

How much of your power is tied up in things you can do nothing about?

What's the total estimated amount of power that's tied up?

STOP now that you know where your power is. There's nothing to fix. Shift gears and go play. You'll bounce off of those things.

Imagine and feel just how powerful and happy you will feel when all hundred watts of your power are available to you. Focus mainly on the state of being you'll enjoy. That's more effective than focusing on the material outcome, and you can begin to enjoy that freer feeling instantly—*right now*.

Can you imagine how magnetic you will be to people, opportunities, and good things when you feel like that? Imagine feeling better and better all the time, feeling better than it's even possible to imagine right now.

Take some time to expand on this, fantasizing pleasantly, light as the touch of a gnat's wing. There is nothing for you to do or fix—just play with this.

Too often we whip ourselves into an emotional state, elaborately imagining and dramatizing things we fear or don't want, yet spend little or no time and energy dramatizing what we desire. Too often we make our fears much more vivid and visceral than our desires. We're awfully good at imagining the scariest and the worst. Think about some of the gut-wrenching Hollywood productions you've dramatized in your head about losses, slights, limitations, hurts, and problems. Those are negative intentions, and they are in the way of your desired outcome.

When was the last time you put on a Technicolor, smell-a-vision, 3D Dolby sound production starring you acting out your heart's desires in vivid detail? Yeah, I thought so.

Imagine the best and prepare to write it down below. It doesn't matter if it comes out exactly like that in reality—it's even best to let go of the fantasy after you imagine it—the point is to find relief and feel better now because it gets you in alignment with your Large Self.

Enjoy this fantasy without grasping at it or needing it to happen on any timetable. Let it go after you're done. There will come a day when you focus like this automatically most of the time. Your mind will be retrained to head toward what you want, no matter what's going on around you. For now, practice!

ACTIVITY: Write out your fantasy in your notebook and take all the space and time you need to flesh out the sensory details. If you can't stick with it, dive deep into the feeling that distracts you from it and drop the story.

Spend more time in elaborate dramatization of what you want
instead of dramatizing scary stories.

* * * * * * * *

The Responsibility Of Big Power

Back when we were first creating our website five years ago, we couldn't help but laugh when I would get so wired or intense or nervous about new technology that felt incomprehensible and out of my control, that I could crash a web server two hundred miles away. That was my first hint that power is a two-edged sword.

More recently, when I was overwhelmed by many giant projects waiting for my attention, someone to whom I had delegated a very important task ignored my instructions and did an astoundingly poor job of it, resulting in thousands of dollars in losses. She'd been causing careless losses and denying it for a while, but I'd kept praising her virtues. Now it was time for a change. When I stepped in, took over, and gave exact instructions, it set her on edge, and tensions that had been building up over her declining work performance for well over a year arose. I didn't say any inappropriate words, but the energy itself was *strong*.

The next day I felt like I had dropped a cluster bomb—*on myself*. Updating some things on the site and still vibrating from that interaction, I crashed an even bigger server thirteen hundred miles away. The host server's tech people could find no logical reason for the crash. Of course not—*I did it*. Some brag they blow things up because they have "big energy"—no—blowing things up is a symptom of big energy *out of alignment*. This crash was a valuable opportunity to bounce off a bad feeling back into alignment, and even got me smiling.

I called the person and we faced the fact that she was no longer enjoying her job. She didn't know how to leave so she'd expressed her unhappiness insidiously. I recognized my counter-intention: dread of the huge task (or so it felt at that time of overwhelm) of finding and training someone else, in addition to all else I had on my plate, and so helped create an increasingly stagnant and negative situation. It began a process that led to letting her go. Everything works out when we make it right. Even pain and conflict can serve us—it might as well once it's there.

As I looked within, intending further insight, the answer was, "As you tap into big power, it becomes even *more* important to watch where you point that thing." As we begin to develop our power of intention, we're wielding a torch, but as we expand it's more akin to an atomic power plant.

Watch where you point that thing.

With big power of intention comes an enormous opportunity to create, light up, and uplift, as exemplified by this note I received yesterday: "I just got an email from Noriko, who shared her Divine Opening experience with you in Ojai the other day (she came from Japan to heal metastasized cancer.) Holy crap, the energy she received must have been huge, because when I read her email and saw her pictures, I was literally flooded with bliss—it felt like it was pouring out of my computer. So thanks for the indirect boost—coupled with the Divine Opening I did two days ago from your book. It took some major blinders off my eyes. Lots of love to you, T"

Power, like gasoline, coal, or any other form of potential energy, is innately neither good nor bad— it's all in how it's used. We bring our own vibration to *it*. Hitler had *big* power. The Presence doesn't judge or withhold.

Stay in balance if you are one who intends very big power. Intend that your heart expansion stays up to speed with your ever-increasing raw power. Intend that your raw power always pass through the softening, tempering vortex of your heart.

On the flip side, spiritual people who are afraid of power for whatever reason don't allow themselves to have much of it, and so never have the impact they could have on their own lives and the world. The extreme of not allowing oneself power is victimhood. Many "good" people are actually pulsing victim energy.

When we do get out of balance, no worries, Life always lines us up with opportunities to come back into alignment; if we're not willing feel that warning, the next one will be stronger. All we need to do is read the Instrument Panel, find a way to make it right, and intend a new, more expanded matrix. The contrast feels so good we want to stay at that new elevation.

* * * * * * * *

Reclaim The Throne Of Your Own Life

Now you're ready to set the intention to claim more of your own innate power. We began this book with the foundational understanding that your greatest power lies in the Non-Physical aspect of you, and that as you put your focus there, your power increases tremendously. Let's do that in a fun, tangible way.

Someone said to me some years ago, "That chair you sit in when you teach is like your throne." I thought about it a minute and it hit me like a lightning strike—of course—I do sit on the throne of my own life in a rather queenly and powerful way! No doubt about it—*I rule my life!*

At the next Five Day Retreat I had everyone sit on that chair, inviting each to experience it as the "Throne Of Their Own Life". It empowered them in a more visceral way than words ever had. Suddenly as they sat on the throne, they could feel it throughout their body. What they had merely known intellectually assimilated deeply and became reality.

You are the Non-Physical king or queen of your domain, complete with your own throne—the Throne Of Your Own Life. Everyone has one, yet you may be letting other people and things usurp *your throne*. Without realizing it you can abdicate your power, forgetting the powerful Non-Physical Large Self you are.

After a while you might begin to feel like it's not even your throne anymore. People may leave it dirty and dented and have no respect for it. They may tell you what you can and cannot do in your own kingdom. You'd like to reclaim your throne, but don't know how.

Here's what you do: kick them all off your Throne. In the privacy of your own mind tell them, "I love you very much, and I allowed you to get up there, but now, *get off my throne—you have one of your own."*

Kick the economy, the climate crisis, your family, friends, peers, work, co-workers, money, anything that worries you, and all your concerns—kick them respectfully off the Throne Of Your Own Life. They don't belong there—you, as your Large Self, belong there.

Your car, your bills, your debt, the healthcare laws, and the government—all those things you put on your throne—kick them respectfully off, making room for you to once again sit on the Throne Of

Your Own Life.

All those concerns you've put on the Throne Of Your Life and given your power are ephemeral. The Non-Physical reality is eternal. It is where your power is. Throw everyone and everything off the Throne Of Your Life so you can sit there calmly or excitedly as you choose, with your Large Self ruling as the sovereign of your reality.

During my first three years of Divine Openings, I kicked absolutely everyone and everything off the Throne Of My Own Life. I went cold turkey, and chose to receive no outside help whatsoever with my emotional, mental, spiritual, and physical health. Having been too dependent on teachers, counselors, books, healers, and seminars in my decades of seeking, and being tired of running on the endless hamster wheel but never getting there, I was serious about becoming completely inner guided, and I was committed to stop giving *any* power away to any outside source; no readings, no sessions, no books or seminars. I made a potent radical decision and stuck to my intention. It worked.

The power I reclaimed was unbelievable. It gave me the capacity to do the work I now do, to help people create miracles, change their lives, heal from illnesses. Walking that talk increases your power as a Conscious Creator exponentially. Living it is where the power is, not reading about it, seeking it, hoping for it, or talking about it. Intending alone isn't enough when it comes to owning your power—it requires following up with firm, consistent actions. I couldn't just say I was claiming all my power, and then run to someone to fix me or clear me.

No one can ever take your power from you, so if they have it, you gave it to them. To build your power of intention, take back power from anyone and anything you gave it to.

People talk about forgiveness, but all it means is taking back the power to feel good—not letting what someone did to you rob you of your joy. Let them off the hook so you can be your Large Self and live a happy life.

ACTIVITY Part 1: Who's On Your Throne?

Ask yourself if you're allowing anyone or anything to occupy the Throne Of Your Life. If you're not, celebrate now! Remember when you reclaimed your throne and contrast the before and after. Yes!

If you've abdicated your throne, who or what's sitting on it now? Anything you give tremendous power to becomes your God. This awareness expands over time. For now just identify the biggest power leaks and intend to stop them. Check if you give power to:

- Your spouse or lover? Your exes—do they still sit on your throne? Take the hit now, feel and experience it fully, and your vibration rises to meet your Large Self. Then there is nothing to fix or heal.
- Your parents and children—take them off the Throne Of Your Life and get *off* their throne! Money—does money have any reality other than what you give to it? Do you spend thoughts and energy on the lack of it? Do you make it your God and let it sit on the Throne Of Your Life?

- The government—do you think laws and regulations control your reality and rule your life? If so, they're on your throne.
- The health-care and insurance systems—do you put them on the throne and give them power over your feeling of well-being and safety? Is fear of failing health on your throne? Is current (temporary) physical reality more real and thus more powerful than your Non-Physical self to you?
- Your healer, teacher (including me—*do NOT give me your power*) psychic, therapist, books, seminars? Do you seek endlessly, trying new paths and processes, thinking the answer it out there?
- Is world peace on your throne? Is your happiness on hold for some day when everyone agrees with you? Who should get to dictate what is correct? Should spiritual and religious people force their versions of Heaven or world peace on everyone else? Would it actually be a good thing if everyone agreed? Would that be a Free Will Universe that honors diversity?
- Corporations—are they on the throne? Do you believe they are somehow limiting your prosperity, or taking something from you, or doing something to you that you and the collective consciousness didn't vibrate into being?
- Your neighbors, co-workers, boss, other drivers on the freeways, taxes, debt, the list is endless. Escort them all off the throne of your life *right now*. And be alert for when you put someone or something back on it!

ACTIVITY Part 2: Make Your List.

Who and what are on the throne of your life, sapping your power, and diluting your intentions?

Write down who and what you give away or leak power to here:

1.

2.

3.

4.

If there are more, write more:

Intend now to move everyone and everything on this list off the Throne Of Your Life. There's nothing to fix—you'll just naturally take your power back and feel better. You don't have to withhold love to reclaim your power. Withholding love feels bad and your Large Self won't go there with you.

Stop judging because it allows you to live and be free.

Summary: Be your Large Self on the Throne Of Your Own Life. Make your choices and actions consistent with that, and your power of intention steadily grows.

Sit On Your Throne

Very consciously play with sitting on the throne of your own life for a couple of weeks or more. You must physically experience this, not just read it and think about it. Designate a big chair or place in your garden as your throne and get out of your head and into your body.

As you sit there for just a few minutes and relax into the silence within, let all of the previous activities where you reclaimed power assimilate and become real in your physical body. On your throne, embody your Non-Physical Self, literally bringing it down to Earth. You'll love all the people to whom you gave power even more because now you won't resent them. You line up with your Large Self as you take back power from any person or thing to which you gave power to hurt, damage, or limit you.

At the next level you're ready to notice how you subtly give power away. For example, it's easy for me to slip into spending too much time working or being busy, and too little simply being with my Large Self. I need a lot of solitude, and my energy drops when I don't take time for it. You may shrink slightly in the presence of certain people, or try to please them. You may fall into other people's habits that don't serve *you*.

Being the master of your own vibration, rather than reacting to other people's energy is essential to building your power of intention. Spiritual people, especially empathic ones, tend to sponge up other people's energy rather than being strongly centered in their own energy. Or they feel others more than they feel themselves and don't know what they're vibrating.

I had to start setting limits on how much I'd visit people to help them in dream state—my sleep was sometimes disturbed and I'd wake fatigued. My unlimited Large Self loves to make those visits, but my physical being is part of that system, and was being affected. I also had to set the intention that any lower vibrations from that went straight to The Void to be recycled and did not stick with me.

When I lead a Five Day Silent Retreat, I must meet the challenge of holding a high vibration, in spite of the fact that the field of resonance of the event is designed to stir the participants up and bring up lower feelings. Being the most powerful component in that atmosphere takes conscious awareness, long baths, deep breathing, and most of all, turning it all over to The Presence. The most powerful energy in the room will dominate.

When you're on the Throne Of Your Own Life, you are the most powerful component in your reality. Others can do what they want, but it doesn't inhibit or limit you. Challenges arise and you simply deal with them, because you're the most powerful component in your life.

Physical Challenges

If there's a problem, I usually don't tell anyone, unless it's someone who can do something about it. You see, when people worry about you, it doesn't help you; their worry vibration can be a counter-intention to your healing, and you don't want that added to the mix. I could feel a mass forming in my breast right after the stress of the old house sale, the move to California, and the fixing up of the new house while trying to keep up with my persistent creative and work drive. It did concern me a bit, but I'm the most powerful component in my life.

I was guided to wait to get healing during the retreat before anything physical escalated. The mass disappeared within days after the retreat, and I got a mammogram to double-check. Without the test I could have told you definitively it was gone, just as I could tell it was there without a test. The decision to double-check in that way was unusual for me, but you can imagine why it was important to check. I have blind spots too, and didn't want to risk having a blind spot cause a big problem. Relief is such a wonderful thing.

Many clients have written to me to say they have healed from something physical after a Divine Opening without asking for a physical healing. They hadn't told me about their physical challenge, but we both got out of the way and The Presence took that opening to heal their physical malady.

It isn't always easy to explain why some people heal physically and others don't. Sometimes they need the illness to spur a change. Sometimes, we're not allowed to intervene. A number of factors can prevent healings. For instance:

- Not feeling worthy of a miracle.
- Not believing miraculous things can happen for them.
- Belief that only doctors can heal illness.
- Belief in the difficulty of healing or the incurability of certain conditions.
- They keep actively regenerating illness with the same vibration, thoughts, and feelings that caused the malady.
- Their Large Self plans for them to transition out of the physical for reasons we don't know.

People have allowed healing of one disorder, then manifested another, indicating one or more of the conditions above. And no one can heal a person who is ready to transition from this physical life back to the Non-Physical.

Consider how you vibrate in your own life. It's more productive to look at yourself rather than others as you practice awareness, because you are in control of you, and you can't create for other people. It's hard for you to read someone else's vibration by looking only at the surface, unless you're a gifted medical intuitive, psychic reader, or a Divine Openings Giver with a gift for reading people, but you can get increasingly good at reading your own vibration.

* * * * * * * *

Play In The Fields Of Intention

When I wish to give a Divine Opening I "do" nothing, send nothing, think nothing, do no process, and am completely passive. My intention causes the Divine Opening to occur, whether the person views a work of art in my book or on the website, or at the end of a course audio. Although the receiver might be on the other side of the world, they often have profound experiences, as powerful as if we were in the same room.

A Divine Opening requires no thought and no action.
It occurs entirely by intention.

I've developed the ability to focus my attention powerfully in such an easy, relaxed and unattached way that a field of resonance is created that entrains other people. It happens as they read my books or sit with me. They begin to vibrate in harmony with this field, and the discordant vibrations they've taken on rise to the level of this very organized field, which affects them, and their entire life, in positive and productive ways.

You could say I help them vibrate who they are so powerfully that the lower vibrations, resistances, distracting thoughts, and counter-intentions that limit them are overwhelmed by the higher vibration of who they really are.

That powerful field of resonance is entraining you
right now, as you read and relax.

It's easy to create such a field of resonance, and you can do it, too. One of the foundational pieces is to master your mind and emotions—which you did or began to do when you read *Things Are Going Great In My Absence*. The unenlightened mind and emotions produce an extraordinary amount of distracting "noise" that ties up energy and contradicts conscious intentions—until the mind is quieted and taken out of the driver's seat and the emotions smooth out.

This book is giving you all the elements you need to master the power of intention, although there is no mechanical process. Think of it as if you're absorbing it all through your skin rather than trying to intellectually figure it out.

The Squirrel In The Tailpipe

One day a friend had a hilarious vision of me in auto-mechanic coveralls, face greasy, one tooth blacked out, explaining how I made the car start. Holding up a dead squirrel by the tail, I say, "Here's your problem right here, missy—there was a squirrel in the tailpipe."

We've gotten so many laughs out of the squirrel in the tailpipe—it's become a running joke, resurrected often. One of us will catch the other off guard with it when talking over what to do about some technical or creative challenge.

In giving customer service, all of us have learned to advise people to "lighten up rather than tighten up," because computers are particularly responsive to emotion and vibration. Sometimes, for no logical reason, someone's computer will not let her log into our site, buy things, or access her course, when there is no problem with the site. There's a squirrel in the tailpipe. We suggest they relax, take a deep breath, take a break and come back later. It usually works. In the office, we also like to say, "That's not real."

Because it's my main mode of communication with my audience and community, when something goes wrong with the website, I can get my vibration out of whack if I'm not mindful. The team has seen me create some really odd phenomena with the website when my vibration about it drops. Someone will look at me, barely able to suppress a grin, and holding up an imaginary limp carcass say, "Here's your problem right here little missy—a dead squirrel in the tailpipe."

Lighten up rather than tighten up.

Commit To Your Large Self

You've known people who date continuously and never commit, and they never get to the richer, deeper parts of relationship. When we meet with The Presence within, it's like finding our soul mate. If we stop dating, appreciate and focus on that love, it grows. But if we keep dating (seeking), our true love is lost. I'm not even talking about commitment to Divine Openings—I'm talking about commitment to your own Large Self—which is exactly what Divine Openings leads you to do.

For one of her shows, Oprah shared her experience in a Tony Robbins seminar. In the exercise in which each person identifies which of the prime human motivations most drives her, Oprah found hers was the motivation to be *significant.* That meant she'd never recognized that *she already was* significant. Insignificance is the same vibration as unworthiness. Tony says if you're motivated to achieve big things and contribute to others *in order to feel your significance,* you are, in his words, "screwed." In spite of all the gurus she knows personally, after spending hours interviewing Eckhart Tolle, after all she's studied, learned, and accomplished, Oprah was still struggling on the personal level—and still seeking her worthiness. Working hard to get worthiness we already *have* by birthright is as pointless as running around spiritually seeking to find what we already have inside.

Oprah has my respect and admiration. I think she would be drawn to the ideas in this book, but Divine Openings or any effective path works best when one slows down and absorbs it deeply rather than running immediately to the next guru or book.

Here's a note from a woman who had the enlightenment experience, and then the contrast of losing it. She attended the Five Day Silent Retreat, had major movement in her life, then got distracted:

> I miss you and Divine Openings! I have stepped off the enlightenment path a bit and got stuck in seekers energy. Geesh, what was I thinking? I know better! Despite this, however, I am moving forward in a beautiful direction.

Seeking is *a lack vibration* more than any particular action. In seeking, there's one of these going on: a paradoxical running from going within, avoidance of feeling or responsibility for one's own vibration, desire to fit in with seeking friends, or even a frantic desperation. Dive into those feelings.

Commit to your Large Self and be faithful to it.

* * * * * * * *

When The Energy Is Too Fast

Without working on myself at all for the past seven years, merely by intending evolution and staying awake as best I can, Divine Openings has expanded me more rapidly than I can sometimes keep up with, and has found its way to over a hundred thirty-five countries at this writing.

If you find yourself over-revved, too buzzed, too hurried, or just not having fun, stop, *intend to assimilate and ground* the energy, smile, breathe into it, and make it right. Smile a tiny smile in your heart. Feeling follows physiology more than you might think. When you smile softly, your mind thinks, "I'm happy." I smile when I'm working out and when doing mundane or boring chores, too.

Divine Openings are accelerators, and if you accelerate your energy faster than you can release resistance to the accelerated Energy / Light / Intelligence, you can get over-revved, and that is not fun. Everything is accelerating at this time, so be sure you're assimilating deeply and grounding the energies before asking for more. Rather than running after a new buzz, slow down and bring it all down to Earth.

In *Things Are Going Great In My Absence* I said you wouldn't need to continue to receive Divine Openings forever to feel better or go higher. Receiving Divine Openings is an awakening, and now, with the touch of a gnat's wing, you can tap into good feelings anytime! You get automatic downloads—feel and live into them.

I don't receive Divine Openings anymore. Even the automatic downloads can get too fast for my physical body/mind if I'm not letting go of the old or releasing resistance to the new, and when that happens I quite simply say, "Slow it down. Help me catch up." Physically grounding activities like gardening, scooping horse poop into a pile, washing dishes, meditating, or walking feel blissfully balancing.

Especially in these accelerated times, we can get pushed to the limits of our ability to expand our pipes, rewire our neurology, and keep up with where our Large Selves are going. We are physical human beings, and while those big accelerating energies are Non-Physical, they permeate and reconfigure your entire being so that you can increasingly *embody* The Presence. That's a tall order. I can handle a lot of energy, but at times, I need a break. More energy is *not* always better. Ask for or allow more energy only when you've grounded and assimilated what you have. If you're scattered, disorganized, or ungrounded, clean up your home and office, sit on the dirt, and land on Earth!

ACTIVITY: Intend To Tap In

Stop right now and tap in. Intend to be your Non-Physical Expanded Self, grounded in your body. Intend to temporarily stop the formation of words in your head. Smile, breathe softly, and appreciate breathing. Notice if you can do it just by intention now!

* * * * * * * *

Your Authentic Self

Seven years ago, as I began to create Divine Openings, my mind thought success would mean being famous, traveling the world constantly to lead seminars, my days filled with sessions, interviews and television appearances, with book after book on the New York Times bestseller list. Earlier in my life—before I knew who I was—I wanted to be a motivational speaker, like Tony Robbins, but now I'm clear I'm not cut out for that.

None of that stuff really suited my talents; in fact, it probably would have made me miserable. As country singer Garth Brooks sang, "Thank God for unanswered prayers." Those were somebody else's stereotypical dreams that wouldn't have brought me the core feelings I wanted: solitude, privacy, and freedom. My authentic style is not to stand on a stage and whip huge groups into a wild frenzy, but to work more quietly at a distance, even in the Non-Physical, and to take smaller groups deeply, quietly into themselves.

It's easy to fantasize about starting a Tony Robbins empire, but when it gets down to true intentions, most people really don't want to do what comes with those fantasies; they just want the *glamour* and wealth they think they would bring.

Rarely have I had visions of where I was going or what it would look like—I've simply followed the trail of what felt good to me and kept refining my own path. Mostly, I've ended up doing things that didn't even exist before, so there was no conventional career path to follow and no degree to prepare me for them. Life brought new and different ways to *feel,* work, and create. I never envisioned my work being Internet based, but my Large Self led me there, and I eventually released my enormous tech resistance. Now I absolutely *love* technology— appreciation for it pulses from me daily.

The blessed Internet is a Godsend that provides me with those core values: solitude, privacy, and freedom, and with the buffer of the website people can't get too attached or dependent on me.

Self-publishing and print-on-demand appeared, setting me free to publish without a big publisher telling me how to write my book and controlling its fate. New share-ware met many of our technical needs. In the office we rave that if we can't find a solution to a need today, someone invents it and it arrives tomorrow or next week.

This beautifully synchronized Universe assembled the perfect components to fit my true, unique heart's desires, building it on that core template of solitude, privacy, and freedom in a way I had never seen it done.

Day by day, the more I expanded into my authentic self, following what felt good to me rather than some stereotypical "form" of success, slowly but surely I discovered what really works for me. It has steadily evolved into a different kind of life than I could have *ever* imagined!

Comparing ourselves to others, wanting what they have, and defining success by other people's models rather than looking inside can rob us of the joy that's uniquely ours. It's waiting for us till we claim it. Paradoxically, one of my famous friends, a sweet guy who was featured in the Secret movie was traveling all the time and experienced health problems from not being able to get himself to say no, or to stop and rest. He told a mutual friend of ours, "I want to do it more like Lola's doing it." He even started recording music after I did! I had to laugh—I used to want to be like famous people—now at least one wants to be more like me!

Discover your authentic self. Your joy is unique.

You might already understand that having lucrative ideas, starting big companies, and making large fortunes provide absolutely no guarantee of happiness. Wealthy people's daily lives still bring challenges, and their relationships are just like yours and mine. You can have just as much or more joy by intending joy.

My intention to have a simple life has clearly kept Divine Openings from getting even bigger. But it's always right where I truly want it to be. There's no struggle between prime intention and counter-intention; I consciously choose the simpler life. One day I might have both the simpler life and the larger organization, but it doesn't matter, I have the *feelings* I want, *now.*

Cultivate the *feeling* you want *now,* and The Presence will guide you to more of that in ways you cannot imagine.

Please note that there is no right or wrong in conflicting intentions. You can have either, both, or whatever you want. Just be conscious and notice if:

- Not risking hurt is stronger than the desire for a relationship.
- Independence and control are more important than a relationship.
- Being right is more important than restoring a relationship.
- Ease, freedom, and comfort are a stronger driving force than bigger success—that's true for me.
- Fear of the new is stronger than desire for something new.
- Resistance to trying new things is stronger than the desire to change.
- Unworthiness is stronger than self-love in making choices.
- Negative attitudes toward money are stronger than the desire to have financial needs and wants fulfilled.
- Fill in your own.

The strongest intention wins.

* * * * * * * *

Amp It Up With Humor

Let's not spend too much time on serious topics and neglect the power of humor, levity, and laughter. I'll treat you to a preview of the first section of my other new book, *Confessions Of A Cowgirl Guru*:

God told me to write this book.

He/She/It did, no kidding. Even told me to call it *Confessions Of A Cowgirl Guru*.

God said: "Lola, you've got more energy than a 1950s housewife on diet pills. Here's another project for you: please, please help bring some levity to the *way* too serious spiritual world. The only people who will talk to me are the spiritual people, and they are so freakin' *serious*. The sinners would be way more fun to talk to but they won't speak to me at all.

"That seriousness is a giant speed bump on the path to enlightenment. Please, tell them it's called en-*light*en-ment, not en-*heavy*-ment. We'd all be having a lot more fun if you guys down there would chill out and just live life. You're running around seeking Me, reading all these books, listening to all those channelers, attending all these seminars, looking everywhere but inside. Hello! I'm right here!"

I agree with God.

Stereotypes are silly to me, too, and it's even more silly when people follow them rather than being who they really are. I don't want to look, sound, act, think, or operate like a stereotypical spiritual teacher, although I am one in a big way, worldwide. Hey, I'm famous in certain small towns where they have nothing better to do.

Humor has added almost as much value to my life as spiritual pursuits, and I rather enjoy defying stereotypes by doing things like writing humor and painting erotic paintings.

My mom said, "You have pictures of naked butts all over your house." I said, "Mom, I know that." She wanted prints.

Penny, a friend of mine, was having lunch with a women's group and someone mentioned my name. Penny kept quiet while they discussed me and noted who had heard of me, until one of them commented with a smirk, "Yeah, Lola Jones. I went to her website. She's like the Marilyn Monroe of spiritual teachers."

My friend Penny said to me, "I don't think she meant it as a compliment, so I piped up, 'Yes, isn't she cool and different? Lola is a close friend of mine!'" The woman changed the subject as Penny grinned hugely.

My love and I like to visit Las Vegas, and that surprises some people. They suspect that on vacation a spiritual teacher would probably visit sacred sites or some crap like that. Oops, that was the cowgirl guru speaking—I would never say crap. But seriously, when you live in nature, beauty, peace, and quiet all the time, where do you go to "get away from it all?"

Sin City! It's so different from my normal life. It's actually quite an amazing place, full of broad contrasts and variety: world-class art, architecture, music, theater, fountains, color, excitement, and prostitutes. Well, I said there were "broad contrasts," and there are certainly all kinds of broads.

I have no interest in visiting sacred sites whatsoever. I live in one all the time and create one anywhere I want to. There's nothing at any sacred site that isn't accessible to me all the time—and you can intend your very own, too. Plus, sacred sites usually have lots of serious people sitting around acting serious or meditating and waiting seriously for Archangel Michael or somebody serious like that to show up—seriously. Given a choice between the sacred and the profane, the profane is more fun, and the sinners laugh a lot more than the saints.

If you ever see me wearing white robes or any kind of Indian garb and speaking in hushed reverent tones, acting pious and spiritual, get a gun (if you happen to be in Texas anybody will loan you one), shoot me on the spot, and throw my body to the coyotes. I am serious. Just this once, I'm serious, but don't expect too much of that from here on out.

Speaking of guns, I've got to tell you that my mother is hilarious; her whole Tennessee-moved-to-Texas family was hilarious, but my mom has the added bonus of being funny when she doesn't know she's being funny—until you start laughing, then she starts laughing. One November, she inquired, "I just don't know what to get you for Christmas, and with you livin' alone out there an' all—would you like a gun?"

She was perfectly serious. I tried to keep a straight face.

I did.

I tried.

"Mom, that is so sweet—so in the spirit of Christmas! I'd think of *you* every time I shot somebody." *Then* she got that was funny, and she laughed. She didn't give up, though. Another Christmas she asked, "Okay, if you don't want a gun, how about a stun gun?"

Had she known that all the houses in the neighborhood had been burglarized, except mine—she wouldn't have been able to sleep. It's been impossible for me to get robbed with the vibration I have.

I rarely even lock my doors, and I've never had an occasion to shoot anyone or even poke a pitchfork at him. In Texas, there's a plaque with a six-shooter on it that some people hang in front of their house that says, "We don't call 911."

Rednecks are fun, though—well, at a distance. We saw another sign on a fence while riding our horses that said, "Caution: Dog can't hold its likker."

Once I told mom about a big health problem I had resolved. She was indignant, "You don't even care enough about me to tell me so I could worry about it?" I started laughing, "Okay, I'm sorry—how horribly thoughtless of me. From now on I will call you immediately if there is anything whatsoever you could be worrying about.

Furthermore, I'm going to turn all my worrying completely over to you, because you—you, my sweet mommy—are a professional."

My Inner Self, God Self, Large Self, Fred, whatever you want to call Him/Her/It is funny, because I asked him/her/it to be. There's nothing worse than an Inner Guiding Voice that only says things like, "Your mission is to save the world," or "You must light a red candle and meditate every day from three a.m. to four a.m."

I've actually woken out of a deep sleep laughing more than once. My Large Self woke me yesterday with this joke: If Divine Openings was an airline it would be called Air Freedom. Our pledge to our customers: "Give us your baggage, and we *WILL lose it.*"

The Presence will happily bring you more humor, levity, lightness, and laughter in your daily life if you ask. I promise you, your Life will overflow with funny people, circumstances, and opportunities to laugh. Appreciate, play it up, and add your own humor.

I'm writing *Confessions Of A Cowgirl Guru* concurrently with this book to balance the seriousness of this book. Life can be joy, or it can be serious. I do my best to set people free from all that, but you were given the precious gift of Free Will, so it's really your choice. Even not choosing is a choice that equals choosing the default option.

Much of *Confessions Of A Cowgirl Guru* was lifted right out of my life experience, but some of it I made up or exaggerated just to amuse myself. Back when I sailed a lot and hung around with sailors, we'd say, "A little varnish is necessary in a good story, as well as on a good boat." In case you have any stereotypes still in place about me, that book will blow them away. Look out! It has cuss words in it! Cowgirls tell it straight up, without candy-assing around.

> *In Confessions Of A Cowgirl Guru I say,*
> *"If you're seekin', you're leakin'." Leaking your power, that is.*

As you know from *Things Are Going Great In My Absence*, I set a powerful intention at one point in my life to cultivate my underdeveloped sense of humor. As a child, if someone teased me, I was humiliated. I was extremely over-serious about myself. That's no longer the case!

If you love to read books, instead of yet another seeking book, read every humor writer and you can find. Some of my laugh-out-loud favorites are the goofy, intelligent writers and comedians such as Dave Barry, Ellen DeGeneres, Bob Newhart, A.J. Jacobs, Craig Shoemaker, Paula Poundstone (and Eddie Izzard on his older DVDs like *Dressed To Kill* and *Definite Article.*)

If you love seminars, instead of yet another spiritual seminar, take a comedy improvisation or stand-up comedy course. A couple of humor instructors once said, "We'll take your dream of making people laugh and turn it into a freaking nightmare." Sounds fun, eh? Take a humor-writing or public-speaking course to improve your communication and timing, as timing is at least half of the effect of humor. My comedic timing gets better all the time, and I am practicing to make a humor DVD.

Watching light-hearted comedy attunes you to that frequency, just like watching crime news, and cruelty attunes you to that. Life is a banquet, and everything is available for those who want it, but you don't have to eat the anchovies off the buffet unless you like them!

My favorite television show is Craig Ferguson's *Late, Late Show*. He has a good time, cracks himself up, and doesn't sweat it. He's smart, and can hold his own with any intellectual guest, but he doesn't take himself or anyone too seriously. I also watch Bill Maher, who is an atheist—he's hilarious. Boy will he be surprised when he dies again. Oh, hello! I love Tina Fey and Alec Baldwin on *30 Rock*. Any chance to read or watch Betty White is a treat for me. Julia Louis Dreyfus as the Vice President of the USA on *VEEP* is fabulously funny. For a list of the humorous and uplifting films I recommend, go to DivineOpenings.com/favorite-movies.

Not realizing it's a choice, too many people live life as if it's terminally serious. And the Universe says, "Yes, right, terminally serious, *terribly* serious—so here are some more terribly, terminally serious things—now you have a lovely matching set."

Our default setting is just to let life happen to us without putting much creative thought into it. Or we can take every opportunity to be silly, smile, laugh, make a joke, intend, enjoy, and make a difference. This is your life, dammit—don't waste it! At the end, what will you say? "I wish I had fretted more about every tragic thing that was happening on Earth," or "I'm so glad I laughed with the people I love."

So many notes have come to us from enlightened people who laughed, soothed, and uplifted their whole family during a parent's last moments, making that parent's transition one of celebration of life, family, joy, and love rather than sadness and loss. One who found Divine Openings and began her awakening just before her mother passed wrote me, "It was the highest quality time I've ever had with my mother."

Intend your life to be full of laughter
and joy, and humor finds you.

* * * * * * * *

Your Words Are Intentions
Or: Watch Your Mouth

"Watch Your Mouth" probably got your attention. When I was a kid, adults would say, "Watch your mouth," if we sassed them or said things they didn't like. Now, you get to watch your own mouth. We throw words around pretty carelessly, and they do matter. Your words don't just describe reality—they create reality.

Grace lifted you as you read *Things Are Going Great In My Absence*, and now all there is to do is make daily choices that make good use of your power. If you choose to jump back in the mud puddle, nose-dive by complaining, deny your power, let your mind run you, work on yourself, or diluting this with New Age junk, Grace simply cannot help you as much, yet will not violate your Free Will.

Being awake requires no work—being conscious is actually fun, empowering, and makes life immeasurably easier. Being unconscious makes life a lot harder and more work. Sometimes people want to do all kinds of processes and complicated magical stuff hoping it will save them from having to think, feel, or choose, and life is all lollipops and flowers—but it all comes down to staying conscious, folks.

The Presence doesn't work at evolution—it's all done by intention—and you can do that too. Of course, the physical realm adds that delicious component of physical work, of gravity, sweat, space and time, so enjoy it, but remember you have Non-Physical power.

Intend to stay awake, aware, and conscious.
It isn't work.

Talking With Others

I'd heard about the traffic in California, but was determined to make the best of it, and have. I never complain about the traffic so my experience of it has been mostly wonderful. Out here, I may check the traffic app before I choose a route, but I don't think about the traffic or talk about it once I'm on the road, even if I hit a slow patch. I think about something constructive, silence my mind and relax, listen to an interesting program, or talk about something uplifting or productive. If I mention traffic, it's something like, "That slow spot wasn't bad at all. I do really well with this overall." Consequently I have smooth trips and am almost always on time. I downplay any exceptions and don't take score!

When you get together with others, be mindful of the conversation if you want to maintain your power of intention. It leaks your power to tell people horror stories of traffic, hassle, failure, victimhood, or what's wrong with this or that. Why point your power of intention at complaints about work, health, injuries, money, or other people, setting yourself up for more to complain about? Of course, others do it, but why sacrifice your power of intention just to fit in?

The sympathy and validation we get from others when we commiserate are a paltry reward considering the high price we pay for it. Before speaking, consider, "Is it uplifting?" "Am I setting myself up vibrationally for more of it in my future?" "Is this building or dumping my power of intention?" Here's the acid test: does it tip your or the listener's nose up or down? That's all that counts!

It might seem that sharing woes and having someone validate our suffering would somehow help, but it doesn't—it literally reinforces victimhood. Smoothly change the subject or tip the nose up if anyone starts to nose-dive the conversation. If it persists, try to exit—life is precious.

Simply trotting out our best intentional speaking when we want to create something doesn't work—our predominant, consistent vibration creates the results. You don't have to be perfect, but think of *everything you speak* as an intention coming out of your mouth, because it is.

Everyday speech affects your power of intention.

Humans tend to want to warn people about things that could befall them, but at best, that's just passing along a disempowering expectation. The people in my neighborhood in Texas tried to warn me about crime, but I just didn't get it. Misfortune, disease, or peril cannot befall a person of higher vibration unless their Large Self is choosing to take them off this planet—and if that's the case, no warning will stop it.

A person attempting to help or warn others should dive into those feelings rather than "sharing" them. If there's a detour in the route they're about to drive, or a hurricane coming, tell them about it, but try not to plant negative expectations.

Humorous tales of woe are particularly sneaky, because we think we're being entertaining, but we're still constructing more of it. Even if we're getting a big laugh, feel which way it takes you and the listener.

No Word Police Required!

There is no need to suffer the Word Police thing, requiring you to carefully say precisely the right spiritual words, prayers, or incantations to have your intention fulfilled. Just be intentional about how your words *feel*.

A friend once told me I needed to say the words *desire* or *choose* and never ever say *want* or *need*. I agree that we must vibrate a light, clear feeling of desire or choice rather than a heavy, lackful, or needy feeling—but it's not the words, it's the vibration! I couldn't say this to her, but things did routinely come faster for me than for her, despite the fact that I was using the "wrong" words and she was using the "right" words.

The difference was our vibration. She was still clinging to blaming others for holding her back. That's a power-of-intention-killer, and using the right words just won't override that vibration. No, you don't need the Word Police—you can talk like a regular person. Just notice the vibration your words create. As you speak, feel it, and notice how you feel and how those listening to you respond. Does vibration rise or fall?

It's particularly annoying to call out The Word Police on other people. Mind your own business and watch your *own* mouth.

Develop Your Power Of Speech

People lean forward to hear what you have to say much more when there's less of it, and when you don't need to be heard.

Now and forever, ask yourself as you talk with people:

- Are my words limiting or negative, i.e. how tough things are?
- Am I talking about nothing?

- Am I talking to avoid silence (PLEASE let the blessed Silence be!) or to avoid going within and talking to The Presence?
- Is it unconscious, "Well, you know how men are, or women are, or kids are, or the economy is?"
- Am I complaining? (Even jokingly complaining is a vibration trasher.) This one is sneaky because EVERYONE DOES IT.
- Am I looking for someone to share and validate my struggles rather than intending to let the struggles go?

A friend who doesn't do Divine Openings asked me for advice about self-publishing—she wanted to write a book about Internet scammers. She's on shaky ground there. It's hard for most people to immerse themselves in a low-vibration subject without attracting that kind of negativity into their own lives. She risks becoming a magnet for scammers, whether on the Internet or when getting her car fixed. We vibrate what we think about, and then attract things that match that vibration. So many of the senators who investigated the porn problem and the preachers who railed vehemently against fornication ended up doing the very things they were fighting against because they were focused on it.

Watch where you point that thing.

- Do I dive into the low vibration within myself instead of "talking about it" which doesn't change it (although I might think it justifies it when others agree how wrong it is)?
- Do I take my joys to others and my low vibrations to The Presence?
- Do I attract people to share and enjoy my chosen reality with?
- Is it uplifting, entertaining, humorous, connective, interesting, heart-opening, or helpful?

Words have power. Use them wisely.

In the Five Day Retreat or other courses when I seem to be just chatting, goofing, sharing, or telling stories, it is never babble. It's always conscious and for a purpose. I try not to complain or speak of limitation much, nor give much energy to what I don't want unless I am guided to say something—I use it to bounce off, toward what I do want. Feel your vibration drop when you complain, gossip, criticize, or speak of lack.

Most people have become so conditioned to put up with things that feel bad, they don't even notice when saying something *plummets their vibration*. But you do. When people have become numb to their Instrument Panel they're mystified, "Where did *that* come from?" They couldn't feel it coming.

The less you say, in general, the more potent it is. If something can be said most powerfully in ten words, saying twenty words dilutes it. If talk is just to fill up empty space, run away from feelings, or distract yourself, stop and feel inside.

Don't dilute the power of your word.

Speaking creates vibrations, and the predominant vibrations create a matrix that is eventually fleshed out and becomes tomorrow's physical reality. Fortunately, you're creating a Non-Physical reality before it pops into physical reality, which gives you a cushion of time to change it if you need to.

Make every word count.

* * * * * * * *

The Best One To Talk To

"Witnessing" is your Large Self observing your small self with wisdom and clarity, without judgment. You get that Larger perspective instead of being stuck inside the smaller, more limited perspective. The witnessing phenomenon of enlightenment happens for some faster than others.

After doing Divine Openings for a while, when you look back at your past, you notice times when you were "in" the drama so much you couldn't see outside it. You were so engulfed in that scenario you couldn't see past it to wider possibilities. You thought those feelings were you, and now from Large Self perspective you know those feelings were just energy moving through you.

The Larger perspective you have when witnessing yourself is always productive, full of possibility, never limited. You hear yourself saying disempowering things in the moment, and you stop immediately.

Witnessing begins to happen automatically at a certain stage of awakening. Intend to witness yourself if you don't already. Listen to your own casual chat. It's actually not *casual*—it's *causal*—it actively constructs!

- Are my words full of possibility, or limitation?
- Am I arguing for unlimited possibility, or justifying my limitations?
- If you hear yourself saying, "Well, realistically . . . ," question it!
- If you hear yourself saying, "There is no way I can . . . ," whoa, there; witness yourself and open up to more of the infinite possibilities your Large Self sees.
- Say, "There are thousands of possibilities when I'm open and feeling good, so I'll focus on feeling a little better and finding my power."
- Say, "I created that, and I can create something else."

Talk is never casual—it's causal.

After you stop thinking of yourself as separate from God, there won't be such a distinction as, "this is me, this is God," or even small self/Large Self. It's just you, relatively more contracted or expanded. Talking to God becomes more like talking to yourself.

Talking to yourself as your God Self focuses you in a powerful, personal, and tangible way on the Non-Physical aspect of you. Talking to The Presence builds your power—do it as you go about your work and leisure, and feel the distinction between you and God disappear.

Make Your Word Mean Business

You are human. You will slip. You will give power away, or you will leak power in subtle ways you may not notice at first. You will sometimes dilute your intentions with contradictory actions.

Re-commit, correct your course, and keep going.

Your situations are probably far subtler than this story, but the counter-intentions and other factors decimating this woman's power of intention make a clear and dramatic example.

I've changed personal details to conceal identity, but the facts are accurate, not exaggerated at all. A woman I've known for a long time is a wonderful, fun, talented, generous, loving person, yet struggles to have what she wants, because she believes she can't have it. She dabbled in Divine Openings but hasn't committed to living it. She says she has the intention of finding a compatible relationship—but she prevents that by staying in a relationship she doesn't want, that is not a vibrational match or a match on any level, out of fear of being on her own financially, and because he's secure in some odd way—he won't leave her.

When the couple met, he didn't feel right to her at all, but he has a vitality that attracted her, he talks big, and is very adoring. She routinely ignores her feelings, so she went full speed ahead. The first week they got together, she fell from a ladder and sustained a double compound fracture. She recognized the message but glazed over, went back to peaceful numbness, and marched on for ten more years and a long string of repeated, regular, serious injuries and car wrecks, many with broken bones—ten or more of them by now. Then a hip surgery. Hips are about moving forward in life—or not. The doctors give her praise for healing fast and rebounding so well, and then there's another injury or wreck. She's ignored her Instrument Panel for so long she doesn't feel any of it coming.

She calls them *accidents*, ignoring that they're Instrument Panel readings escalated to fire-alarm intensity. *There are no accidents, only messages.* Even if accidents did exist, the statistical probability of anyone having as many disasters in nine years as she has had is nil.

Her injuries mirror her hurting *herself,* but in calling them *accidents* she casts herself as a powerless *victim* of random events, giving away her power as a Conscious Creator. The moment we say, "I created that," we begin to get our power back.

For ten years, she's said she wants out of the relationship. Once, eight years in, she said to her partner, "I'll let you live here as a roommate to help me out with rent. We are not a couple," but he ignored her and continued to talk and act like her partner, because her word on this subject means absolutely zero. She lost even more power.

Actions speak louder than words.

Over the years, I'd say things she could not yet hear. Lovely person that she is, she never got defensive—she'd just smile and march on to the next disaster. Our job is simply to love people like her, and let them have their Free Will choices.

By acting as if this man is her financial hope and security, she pinched off her own money flow. After each injury she had no income, because her work is very physical. The man contributes very little money, and the medical and other bills became substantial. She had to declare bankruptcy.

Her intentions were split:

1. Prime intention - have a great relationship and life.
2. Counter-intention – be adored by someone who will never leave, get half the rent paid each month, comfort zone, illusion of security.

Recently, she was vibrationally able to hear it, so I asked if she wanted input and she said, "Yes!" I offered, "For our words to wield great power we must match what we do with what we speak. *Everyone,* including the Universe, believes the actions, not the words. With decades of practice doing things that feel bad to you while numbing yourself to the feelings, Life has to scream at you with escalated *events.* When you continue to ignore your feelings, the signals get really radical. Resistance is supposed to feel worse and worse so you'll stop it. You're not supposed to get tougher and better at withstanding the disasters!"

She was finally willing to see the *accidents* as Instrument Panel readings, and see that the financial and security counter-intentions had actually cost her far more than she gained. When we sell ourselves out, we always pay for it in other ways.

Doing *things that don't feel good to* us is the most damaging thing we can do. It *should* feel like self-abuse. It should set off all kinds of alarm bells. But people who have been ignoring their feelings for decades are *so numb* it just feels *normal* to them. This woman's relationship, money, and health were all out of alignment because she did not listen to or act upon her own feelings.

By making any person or thing our savior, our relationship with The Presence becomes weak— when it's strong, we go within for all those needs. One could own up and say, "I've been making this person my God and my security, so my relationship with God is weak. I'm responsible for the fact that my words have come to mean nothing. I've put my future in *this other human's hands,* instead of in God's hands.

Her future hung in the balance. If she reclaimed the power of her word and her power of intention, there would be a cascade of positive events. It she didn't, her power would weaken even further, and *escalated* disasters could be expected. This story has a happy ending. She found the courage to listen to herself and end the relationship. She feels honest, free, and powerful, although there were some moments of panic at first.

When your words mean business,
your power of intention increases.

Secondary Gain

Some counter-intentions offer no benefit—they are simply limitations, fears, or lower vibrational beliefs. But some counter-intentions offer a "secondary gain"—a payoff that sweetens up the allure of the counter-intention.

You'd think that abandoning one's true desires to settle for a limiting counter-intention would not be attractive, but the woman in the story above is *getting a paltry payoff—she* gets to stay in an odd kind of comfort zone. To her, at least that comfort zone is guaranteed, real, and it's here now, while her prime intention seems out of reach or even impossible. The meager payoff, however small, of that comfort zone is easy for her to rely on, so she takes that tiny payoff instead of going for her prime intention.

Because perception is reality, it doesn't matter if the payoff is imaginary or real. The meager, reliable, here-and-now good feelings this man gives her may seem not worth the price she's paid, but she imagines them as more real than the promise of an ideal compatible partner she's never had.

The counter-intention, with its paltry secondary gain payoff, is nevertheless winning, because our "action vote" counts the most.

People who smoke get the secondary gain of numbing their feelings so they don't have to deal with them. They get instant, if only temporary relief. If they feel concern for the long-term effects, they smoke another cigarette, and presto, that feeling is gone too. People using food or other substances for relief or a treat are getting a secondary gain of feeling a tiny bit better instantly, without having to change, face their own resistance, or feel those lower vibrations they're trying to escape.

Even if the secondary gain is paltry and fleeting relief, it's easy to keep doing it simply because it is a habit. Habits are by definition self-perpetuating. Sometimes this is good—you don't have to think about driving your car—it's a habit that runs automatically. But when the habit is an addiction, it takes over the person's Free Will and uses their power for its own purposes, and it only has one purpose—to maintain the habit. Addiction prohibits us from looking for better ways to find relief and live more fully.

Use the extreme examples I've given you to bust any subtle counter-intentions (some supported by secondary gains) that you might have.

Support your spoken intentions
with matching vibration and action.

Reclaim your power without judgment or self-blame:

> *I am saying one thing and doing another—my intentions are split.*
>
> *I created that by default or counter-intention.*
>
> *I reclaim my power by following through on my words.*

Power of intention increases dramatically when vibration, words, and actions are consistent, but people often call us "lucky." We're not lucky. When we speak it, it will work out in some way eventually. When we're not committed to action, we just don't say it, except in a brainstorming context where we're just tossing out ideas.

Every day you choose a fork in the road that either honors your word and supports your stated intention, or it doesn't.

It's obviously not about being good or doing the "right thing," it's about the difference between being powerful or dumping power. Being honest with yourself increases your power of intention.

If I find I can't do what I said I'd do, I say so—then there's no power loss. If I can't keep a commitment, I own it, apologize, clean it up, and resolve it the best I can, without rationalizations or excuses.

Excuses and rationalization drain power by claiming that outside forces determine what happens to and for you. I'd rather say, "I created it" than be a powerless victim of circumstances and events.

These are power-dumping rationalizations and the corrected power-claiming statements:

I am behind because . . .	I'm behind because I didn't manage time.
They or it limit me.	I'm limiting myself.
I can't because . . .	I don't want to.
The reason I didn't do it is . . .	I just didn't get it done.
Someone else is at fault . . .	I created that.

Live your commitments. Claim your power. Keep gently throwing other people and things off the throne. Some things are really sneaky and you'll put them on the throne and not notice. No worries—your Instrument Panel will read low, it will feel bad, and that will get your attention. Then you'll get back on the Throne Of Your Own Life.

* * * * * * * *

Is It Patience Or Resistance?

Observing people is interesting. I've watched some acquaintances say, very spiritually, that they're being "patient" about living into their intentions, and then I've watch them be patient—for another ten years—and their intention is still not happening. That is not patience; that is a spiritual bypass, smiling and pretending it's okay, ignoring that it's not moving, and not doing anything to release the resistance. Neither The Presence nor I am judging; it's no crime to hold yourself back. This is just to say that if you've been "patient" for a very long time, wake up. The Presence fulfilled your desire and started the party very quickly. Where are you?

Turn Drama To Excitement

One client was unconsciously creating high drama in her life, and through Divine Openings, she saw it was due to not letting herself have the high-excitement music career she once had and really wanted again. Her counter-intention was that she always had to know all the answers before beginning an endeavor, and so avoid risks. Once she began taking healthy steps toward doing her music, the unhealthy drama abated.

If we need more excitement and don't create it consciously, we can default to drama to spice things up. Affairs, unexpected expenses, injuries, losses, and all kinds of drama befall those who aren't giving themselves a needed change or enough positive excitement. There are no accidents.

Drama is addictive to the system. People addicted to drama, risk-taking, or abuse, create terrible things they swear they don't want. Drama certainly makes one feel alive in an edgy way, but you, powerful Conscious Creator, can choose more productive *and* enjoyable ways to feel deliciously alive!

Serial seekers use their "issues" and exaggerated emotional processing to keep life dramatic and get attention. Others use crazy romances, office politics, or gossip to get their fix. Drama is a poor-quality buzz compared to positive excitement.

The choice is: create drama by counter-intention, or deliberately intend positive, challenging excitement.

ACTIVITY: Do You Want Excitement Or Drama?

Check your life: are you creating challenge, excitement, and interesting things to experience on purpose? Are you hanging out with fun people who have healthy adventure in their lives, who are doing productive things and having real fun?

Or do you find yourself in dramas you didn't notice you were creating? Are you hanging out with drama queens? If you are, chances are you're a vibrational match to them; otherwise you'd find it unpleasant and gravitate away. If you truly don't enjoy drama, you attract others who don't.

Intend to be done with drama. Intend the feelings of excitement or newness or exploration that you want and let go to them. Imagine the feeling of having fun and adventure without drama. Then you won't let that sneaky counter-intention attract drama into your life by surprise.

Follow-Through Power

Everyone gets excited when they get a new idea or desire. The Non-Physical "whoosh" of energy and the resulting physical high of something new being conceived is universal. The contrast as it sweeps you upward is like an exciting amusement park ride. It's the easiest part of any creation.

Dreaming of a baby to love is thrilling, and most would agree that conceiving a baby is the easiest and most fun part. Then there's the follow-through: getting up at all hours to feed the baby, changing diapers, bathing, rocking, protecting, dressing, and minding the baby.

Most would agree that the first blush of new love is the most heart-palpitating part of a relationship. After the high of the honeymoon comes the follow-through: adjusting to living together, divvying up chores and responsibilities, paying the bills, maintaining the house, and earning and deciding how to spend income. Casanovas love starting new relationships but not the follow-through—preferring the thrill of the new.

When you set an intention or have a new idea, you get that big rush. You're playing the first of three roles in getting a new creation out to the world: the role of the "starter." Sometimes starters follow through on the intention and take it all the way to physical materialization and sometimes they don't. Some lose interest as the newness and the rush fade.

Sometimes the excitement *should* fade. Play with your idea and let it mature a while before you commit too many resources. Often an idea blossoms into a better idea or leads you down several trails to the best path of all.

Let's say one day you intend "time freedom," and the very next day you're shown an exciting business that would absolutely make you rich. Luxuriate in the "time freedom" feeling you want for a while, and let The Divine parade more options by you. Allow yourself to enjoy the excitement of all these new ideas, but eventually choose the one that most matches that feeling of "time freedom." That first lucrative, attractive idea may leave you far less free time than you wanted, and if you don't get that feeling you wanted, no amount of money can replace it. You may eventually choose less money, more time, or you may get both, but you'll be happy, and that's what counts. I have numerous ideas every week that I reject for just such reasons.

Once you've chosen the *best idea of the lot,* the one that will give you most of the feelings you want, follow through and take it to materialization. It takes maturity and commitment to follow through. Yet another new idea distracts some incredibly creative and talented serial-starters before anything materializes with the previous idea, because the rush of starting is more exciting than the follow through. Ideas, without plain old mundane, non-glamorous follow-through, die young.

Creations must be promoted and taken out in the world to complete the follow-through—or they die at that late stage. People without high *follow-through power* don't do well in self-employment unless they work with others who do have it.

Before we go into how to intend more follow-through power, there is no rule that says you must follow through at all. The Presence doesn't judge. If you choose not to follow through on your ideas, that's fine—just be conscious about your choices, and say, "I enjoyed the whoosh of the idea and that's all I want for now." Then you don't lose your power of intention.

Rather than splitting your energy by saying you intend to do something when you have stronger counter-intentions and indeed will not do it, intend to fully enjoy your ideas as pure Non-Physical creations and don't torture yourself. Stop resisting your resistance, which just might help you materialize it more easily at some future date when you're more ready for it!

Be satisfied with being a dreamer and enjoy your rich inner life. You get the thrill of creation, and the good feeling doing it would have brought you—without doing anything! Don't reverse that great feeling by making yourself wrong for not following through. Remember, it's the feeling you wanted in the first place. But if you truly want those dreams to materialize, follow through.

Consciousness is all-connected, and there are many documented cases where inventions or scientific concepts were conceived simultaneously by several people in distant parts of the world. You've probably seen some of your ideas in television ads and said, "Darn it, they stole my idea!" No—they had that idea too, but followed through—if you don't, someone else will.

I'll often say something new or in a way I've never said before, and Esther Hicks channeling Abraham will say the same thing the next week, or vice versa. We're all sparks of God, so, of course, we have some of the same ideas.

There are unlimited ways to get things done and make money even if you intend to remain exclusively a starter. Put it on the God list and be alert for answers, but here are a few ideas:

- Hire finishers and maintainers, but your energy and intention are still required until the stage when you can turn it over to them.
- Inspire volunteers to do it for you but, as above, you're still critically involved.
- Sell your ideas.
- Write them into fictional entertainment—Jules Vern never built a rocket, but inspired others to do so.
- Assemble a team with all the elements you don't have.
- Work for a company that supports you, provides a steady paycheck and a follow-through structure with deadlines, and do your piece of its work. You can contribute bright ideas that add value.
- Open your pipes enough to let in money without working.
- If you truly want to increase your own follow-through power, bust your counter-intentions.

Sample counter-intentions in italics:

- I get excited about ideas, but *don't inject joy into the mundane work.*
- I want change in my life but *don't want to change.*
- I want something new but *want my old comfort zone more.*
- I want to do something but *don't want the responsibility or risk.*
- *My fears are stronger* than my desire for the new thing.
- *I don't believe I can* do, be, or have that.
- *I'm not willing to do it badly* in order to learn to do it well.
- *I must be perfect at the start* or I won't take the journey.
- *I don't tolerate risk* but I want to be self-employed.
- *I can't self-promote* but I want exposure of my gifts.
- *I prefer a paycheck that arrives on time every week* (there is fine unless you truly want to be self-employed.)
- *I let excuses or mental noise drain energy* I could use to take action.
- *I let resistance stop me* and then I don't resume.

Starter energy conceives ideas and sometimes launches them. Follow-through energy takes it all the way to materialization and success. Follow-through energy helps you enjoy the challenges of learning new things and overcoming obstacles as you get the idea out to the world and in the hands of those who can benefit from it.

Some people move all the way through starting and follow-through into the third and final role: "maintainer." Maintainer energy keeps the project going successfully long-term, through many years. Maintainers are usually dependable, steady focusers. Strong maintainers are tolerant of sameness and need less radical change—they find perpetuating and nurturing the status quo quite fulfilling.

Different personality types excel at different stages.

You can intend to develop all three skills: starter, follow-through, and maintainer. To see which you now *tend toward,* look at your life. Starters love new things. Some starters take many of their ideas to materialization. Other starters fizzle after the thrill of the idea fades; or they start work on a project but don't follow through; or at the first challenge, they drop it and start an exciting new project, which also may not get out to the world.

Those with follow-through power don't stop until success is accomplished, even if they have to change course repeatedly. Working for themselves or others, they do or delegate the many steps to take an idea to completion, which includes getting it out to the world. They release resistance and step out of comfort zones. They manage or even relish the learning curve, mastering all the many skills they need to get something done. They may learn to collaborate, market, write, make videos, promote themselves, make sales, manage people, or develop a hundred other skills, including ones they didn't have before.

Classic maintainers might create their own idea and take it all the way through to the maintaining stage; or they may go to work for starter and follow-through people and do the maintaining for them, or purchase a starters' idea or a follow-through person's well-designed franchise and run it successfully long-term. They typically can happily stick with the same winning formulas over time, and require less change.

Starter power, follow-through power, and
maintenance power are all important.

Those who accomplish the most either cultivate a balance of starting, following through, and maintaining, or they get others to do the parts they don't do as well.

Entrepreneurs can face a critical point when a business reaches a pinnacle of success, perhaps the day the business reaches a long-desired goal. For some, having climbed the mountain and reached the summit, there's suddenly no more challenge and the thrill is gone. The entrepreneur might sell that company to a maintainer who'll run it successfully for life.

Some people with high need for newness keep it fresh by continuing to create new things within the old container. I must always be creating something new, but there's always careful attention to follow-through, and maintaining past creations, nurturing, enlivening, and improving them. Intention and attention keep all my work vital and alive. That's my maintaining energy.

I will die with a long to-do list still undone and all those creative desires will keep me vital and alive until then. If you like doing many things, as I do, the variety gives rich contrasts and offers a break from one thing while doing another. But occasionally, as with this book, I needed to stop spreading my time too thin, ignore the long to- do list, and follow through and finish just this one thing. No one can truly multi-task—that's actually just jumping from one thing to another sequentially.

Know yourself. I'd never be a great opera or rock singer, but I do well with jazz and pop. I'm not a great accountant. I manage my organization well, but I'm not an ambitious, empire-building type, so I don't ever wish for that.

To increase follow-through and maintaining power:

- Thinking about doing it takes *far more energy* than actually doing it.
- Resisting a task takes *far more energy* than actually doing it.
- It's never as bad as the wrong-seeking-missile-mind imagines.
- EQ: *How great will it feel when it's done?* Focus on the feeling you'll get on a task's completion instead of how hard or tedious it is to do it. I do this with all activities I don't like: filing, paperwork, taxes, and learning new technical things.

When you first dreamed up the business or the relationship you were focused on how good it would feel. If you lose the thrill when faced with the daily mundane tasks, go back to *how good it felt.*

Focus on how great it will feel when it's done.

High Payoff Activities

Having been successfully self-employed most of my life, I've learned that if what I'm doing supports me, I get to keep doing it. I've also learned that I could be "busy" all day, and be tired at the end of the day, but if I was busy with *low payoff activities* or *no payoff activities* there simply was no paycheck. This one powerful idea can revolutionize your results in any endeavor:

Each day, do the Highest Payoff Activities (HPA's) first.

If you want a business, project, or dream to succeed, apply most of your time and focus to High Payoff Activities—activities that produce profit so you can keep doing what you want to do.

If your goal is a steady job, searching employment sites on the Internet is not an HPA—calling to get an interview is an HPA. Refining your resume is not HPA—going on an interview is an HPA. If you're a consultant, improving your website is fun, but it's not an HPA—driving traffic to your site or meeting potential clients at networking meetings is an HPA. For the artist or musician, painting or writing music is absolutely necessary, but the Highest Payoff Activity is getting it seen and heard out in the world so it can create financial support.

People often avoid their HPA's because of resistances: inertia, fear of the unfamiliar, risk, rejection, and resistance to doing challenging tasks. Sure, busy work and low payoff activities are usually easier—they're good for a short morning warm-up, but not sufficient to support you. Evaluate your to-do lists carefully, and rewrite them with your HPA's at the top. My to-do list is called the God List, because I turn it over to The Presence before I take any action, and lots of it gets done in easier ways than I expected, and some gets done without me.

High Payoff Activities are a big key to success.

If you need immediate income, find short-term High Payoff Activities that produce faster results, then add long range High Payoff Activities. Sometimes, taking another short-term job keeps your vibration up while your next plan is developing.

Summary:

- Once that biggest rush from the birth of the idea has faded, find ways to enjoy the follow-through.
- Focus on the feelings you want from completion.
- Chunk it down into small steps. Do small steps each day.
- Identify and do the Highest Payoff Activities first every single day.
- Generate energy. En-joy means *put the joy into.*
- Enjoy the ride as you gain the skills and knowledge you'll need. .
- Tell yourself supportive stories—you're making it up!
- Celebrate and take score of each small success.
- Stay flexible on the specifics and the *form* things must take. Let Life lead you to the next step.
- Let feedback and failures guide you, but don't take score.
- Let The Divine do the heavy lifting—put it on the God List.
- Let in help!

There are several audios in the Level Two Online Retreat in which I coach people on HPA's, along with many other topics and fun activities not included in any of my books. I love the flexibility of the online retreats because I can continue to add to them long after the books are finalized and published.

* * * * * * * *

Chunk It Down

How do you build a house? One brick at a time. A big project can feel impossible, but one small chunk each day feels entirely doable. Chunk your projects down into very small steps. Put the whole thing on the God List, *but take a small step each day, starting today*. That jump-start beats inertia. Now you're rolling—continue to do steps one at a time.

Resistance eats far more energy than doing the task!

"Becoming a rock star" is too large a chunk. Taking a series of guitar lessons is a manageable chunk. Auditioning one band member is a small chunk. Practicing regularly is a series of small chunks. Learning how to book yourself for gigs or finding a manager is another small chunk. Your first gig is a small chunk. Raising money to record a CD is a series of small chunks. Then, Grace kicks in and follows your lead, fleshing out your matrix, adding bricks—or sending bricklayers to help.

Chunk it down and resistance reduces.

Small-chunk details can get you lost in the story if your vibration is low. If that happens, jump back up to the big picture and focus on how you want it all to *feel*, what you love about what you're doing, and what's right in your life. Soothe yourself with big picture thoughts like, "I am cultivating the feeling of freedom," "Things always work out," "I have many things going for me to feel good about right now," "I know how to rise up the Instrument Panel," "A big journey is made of many steps, and I don't have to know it all now."

Stay in the big picture while raising your vibration. Go back to focusing on detailed chunks when you're feeling good.

Never let yourself stay in a low vibration for too long.

Generate Energy To Break Through Inertia

A common factor with people who take ideas, desires, projects, dreams, or companies through to materialization is they *generate* their own energy rather than waiting for it to magically *appear*. They rave, rev it up, and *inject* power into it. When I sit down I can always write. I don't know what writer's block is because I generate energy, reality, and creativity rather than waiting for it to fall on my head.

If there's resistance, powerfully intend it to move, and know when to take action and let momentum overcome resistance, or wait a bit. Don't wait forever, though. Focus and take one small step, zapping the biggest barrier to all progress—inertia.

Inertia is a law of physics that says a body at rest
tends to stay at rest, and a body in motion tends to stay in motion.

Inertia, like gravity, just is—there's no right or wrong about it—we just learn how to deal with it. Once you focus, *smile,* and begin, momentum accelerates, your Large Self takes over, and then inertia is on your side. Once you're moving, you tend to keep moving.

Give It Over Or Give Up

It may seem odd to talk about following through and then say, "Give it over or give up." Yet it's pretty simple: if you're in the flow, pulsing as your Large Self, follow through with details and action, and en-joy it. If you're not clear and vibration is low, give it over to The Presence, take a break, and get out of the way.

You already know that when you give something big over to The Presence, you relax, breathe a sigh of relief—you feel a heavy weight lifted right off your shoulders. Even if you're feeling good, it's wise to give it over from the start if it's too big for you to do alone, whether it's finding a relationship, reaching enlightenment, getting into an exclusive school, realizing a big creative dream, or paying off a huge debt.

You've read the notes and maybe heard the audios from the people who struggled and strived for liberation on the spiritual path, asking question after question, reading book after book, trying to figure it out mentally. They come to Divine Openings and yet still drag that old work-on-it paradigm into this. Then, one day they let go and it just happens. They finally get out of the way enough to allow it in.

When you give it over to The Presence, or put it on the God list and let go, you're suddenly not fretting, tensing, and resisting. You may not be perfectly aligned but you're not in the way anymore. New insights and possibilities come to you, or the situation resolves itself.

Your intentions are most quickly realized from a state high on the Instrument Panel. You might argue, "Then how can people have miracles happen when they're in crisis, grief, or devastation?" In counseling thousands of people, and in my own experience, I find it's actually at the point where the person in difficulty "gives up" or takes even a brief break from stress that the miracle happens. When you give up, you stop struggling and you relax for a moment, and "Boom!" there's a crack of an opening for Grace to help you.

Two women each told me how they avoided a car crash that was inevitable and logically impossible to prevent. Dinorah, a Divine Openings Giver in Stockton, California, was driving along when another car ran a stop sign and headed right toward her at high speed. It was going to hit her broadside. But then, she found herself on the other side of the intersection, and miraculously, impossibly, the car didn't even touch her car. She has no idea how it happened. In the same situation, another woman, Shirley, closed her eyes, took her hands off the steering wheel, and let go. Her vehicle flew through the intersection, missing many solid obstacles, and came to a stop safely. *Then* she opened her eyes.

When we galloped, Casanova, a beautiful but crazy horse I once owned, would sometimes put his head up in the air, brace against the bit, and refuse to stop. One day he desperately wanted to get back to the other horses who were on the other side of a ditch filled with giant, angular boulders, each about three or four feet square. I wouldn't have wanted to try to pick through those boulders on foot. There were jagged gaps between them and their steep, slick sides offered no traction.

The only safe way to get back to the other horses would have been to go around the ditch, but Casanova was out of his mind—with his head in the air he couldn't see where he was going and we were racing toward the ditch at a full gallop.

While my mind was alarmed in a rational way, at some point I gave up. Mere yards from the ditch, a sense of peace came over me, and I let go, turned inward, and blinked my eyes slowly. In a nanosecond we were somehow past it. Impossibly, there was no stumbling or clattering of hooves, there was no leap into the air over it. There was just an inexplicably smooth arrival on the other side. I'll never forget it. Whether you let go deliberately, or just plain *give up,* you're suddenly out of the way.

How to get out of the way if it's too big for your human self:

- Focus on the powerful and vast Non-Physical You rather than on the physical you.
- Put it on the God List, then . . .
    - Give it over to The Presence and take yourself off the case.
    - Prostrate (it's in *Things Are Going Great In My Absence.*)
    - Take a break and go have fun to feel better.
    - Give up—stomp or throw your hands up in the air and quit.
    - Take a short "time out" from thinking about it and acting on it.
    - Dive in (it's in *Things Are Going Great In My Absence.*)
    - Go to The Void (we'll cover this soon.)

Soon after the incident with the ditch, I received guidance that I had just about punched my ticket with Casanova and that I needed to take some conscious action, give him up entirely, and get a safer horse. Casanova had fulfilled a counter-intention to create drama and excitement and impress my friends with my cowgirl fearlessness and riding ability—I was done with that.

Grace keeps saving you up to a point, but then The Presence says, "Hey, how about if you do your part and quit throwing yourself in front of trains." My next horse Royal, who is still with me after ten years, is just spunky enough to be exciting without being either dangerous or boring.

ACTIVITY: Grace does its part. Do your part.

Is there a situation in your life where Grace has repeatedly saved you, but now it's time to evolve, be conscious, and make intentional choices? Is it with your health, eating habits, an unhealthy relationship, a child, an addiction, a living situation, or something else?

* * * * * * * *

From Devil's Choice To New Possibilities

Humans sometimes give themselves a Devil's Choice. A Devil's choice gives you *only two* options—and neither one is satisfactory. It goes like this: the devil welcomes us to Hell (if the devil or hell actually existed) and says, "You can sit on those hot coals, or you can sit on these sharp spikes. Your choice." The devil's choice is no choice at all.

We don't have to choose either one! Devil's Choices come from buying into limiting, disempowering beliefs. There are other, better choices outside of that reality, like leaving hell, which most of you have done!

Who made up this "only two choices" thing? The mind loves opposites and polarities. Black or white, us or them, work or play, this or that.

Now that your awakening has begun, your Devil's Choices are probably subtle and sneaky:

> *"I can tell the truth and suffer for it, or lie and save face."*

> *"I can honor my feelings and risk someone not liking it, or repress my needs and avoid conflict."*

> *"I can eat all the junk food I want and be fat and happy, or eat boring, healthy food and have no fun."*

Since perception is reality, if you buy into the devil's choice it feels as if there are only two choices available to you in the whole Universe, and that's never true.

Outside the Devil's Choice lies *unlimited possibility*. You don't have to accept A or B—you can create something you didn't even know was possible. When I catch myself buying into a Devil's Choice, I say, "Rewind!" then ask myself an Effective Question (EQ), "What are the many options beyond these two?"

Some Devil's Choices tell you two great things are mutually exclusive and you can't have both, when you could actually *have both:*

> *"I can leave this man who dominates me and be free, or I can stay and be repressed."* You can change your own vibration and he can't dominate you anymore. You could fall back in love and stay.

> *"I can be assertive and get respect, or I can be nice and be liked."* You can grow a spine and people will love you even when you disagree or say tough things that need to be said.

> *"I can skip this year's vacation and pay off my debt, or take a vacation and go deeper into debt."* Or you can take the vacation and get so much relief and clarity you make more money to pay off your debt when you return. Or you can get paid to go somewhere on vacation. There are millions of choices when you're being your Large Self.

A man meditates and blisses out all the time but is frustrated because it's impossible to work and pay the rent while living the deep spiritual life he wants. A woman wants to quit her corporate job, thinking it's "selling her soul"—mere perceptions that create a reality.

Rather than trying to figure it out in the physical realm, just intend the *feelings* you want from both of the seemingly warring intentions: bliss about the spiritual life *and* the security of having the rent paid. Security and comfortable support of the corporate job *and* a fulfilled life.

The next section offers you a way to create new things when you have no idea what you want, how to find it, or how to get there!

Perception is reality, so if you think the
devil's choice is real, it is.

* * * * * * * *

Ask Effective Questions

In the old paradigm, we asked other people, traditions, experts, or texts for *answers*, seeking reassurance, safety, or known facts to rely on.

At this level of Divine Openings we ask our Large Selves directly, to *open up new possibilities*. Effective Questions (EQ's) point your consciousness in productive new directions, not to fix anything, but to create something new—just because you can.

Here are some examples of Effective Questions:

What if you had a powerful way to turn negatives to positives?

How would it feel to create more results with less work?

What if you could tip the nose up without resistance from your mind?

Notice how just asking these Effective Questions causes your mind to get curious and expand your sense of possibility, even though you may not get immediate answers.

EQ's help you let go, which allows your Large Self to bring you higher vibration possibilities even beyond currently known facts and resources. You don't let your limited mind answer the questions—your Large Self answers them. It may sound like your voice answering as your Large Self puts the words in your mouth; or you may hear nothing, and the new possibilities simply play out in your life as the stepping-stones appear in front of your feet.

Just asking an EQ changes your vibrational state. You move gently into the big picture, full of curiosity and possibility rather than sorting through the overwhelming details and facts. You relax knowing you don't have to find the answers yourself, argue with your limitations head on, or decide right now.

EQ's Are Forward Focused

EQ's point you forward into the fresh and new:

What is possible that I haven't thought of or done before?

How can I have something better than this devil's choice offers?

Who knows something useful about this?

What will my life be like when I have enough money?

When people tell me they don't see "how" they can pay off their debt or revitalize their relationships, I say, "The *details* of "how" are not your job." Ask some EQ's, let go, and it's your Large Self's job to go after the answers. Just keep your nose tipped up and focused on the *big picture* of how you want to feel. Be ready to move your feet when you get the urge.

EQ's are *useful questions* that instantly *give you relief.* They playfully, gently open up possibilities and help you let go of details that limit you.

EQ's often begin with "What . . ." and "How . . ."

Remember that at the beginning of the book I asked my Large Self, *"What makes power of intention stronger or weaker?"* That was an Effective Question! I've created such a habit of asking them I do it automatically now. I ask, let go, and my Large Self downloads the answers at some point, and this time surprised me with the detail and specificity. It would have been too much all at once! I wouldn't have been able to type that fast. Remember this if you think you need all the answers or the master plan at once—be glad it doesn't come that way.

As a full-time corporate consultant and trainer in the 1990s, Effective Questions were one of my most powerful tools, because the mind is helpless to resist them. Even extremely resistant minds can be led with EQ's because they broaden the mind, distract it from details, facts, and problems, tempting it to get curious about other, larger possibilities.

Because I had already mastered EQ's, I was hired on a team that trained managers all over the country at GMAC Finance, a division of General Motors. Managers were able to stimulate more resourceful, proactive thinking from themselves and their employees, and that division became their most profitable, even as the rest of GM struggled. Then, I developed a new and improved course using deeper principles that later became part of Divine Openings, and taught it at IBM and many other companies.

Long before Divine Openings I was using EQ's to help people lead more powerful meetings, coach employees, engage teams, be more influential, make more sales, and much more. They'd come back with touching stories about using EQ's at home, sharing how family issues resolved as resistance melted. You'll be able to use EQ's to tip the nose up, retrain your mind to open up to Grace, and create with more ease. You'll love using EQ's to lead your mind rather than letting it lead you.

If you say to someone, "I know a better way to do this," it may set up resistance. If you say, "How could this be easier for you?" doors open.

If you're worried, and you tell yourself, "Stop worrying! It will be all right!" it may create more resistance. If you say, "What solution could I come up with that I haven't thought of yet?" resistance softens. Effective Questions gently tease the mind into opening to new possibilities rather than smashing head-on into its resistance.

We ask ourselves an Effective Question, relax, and let our Large Selves bring the answers. The answers don't always come in words—but as feelings rising, doors opening, situations shifting, or resources materializing.

Use Effective Questions to create new possibilities
in the Non-Physical first.

EQ's get your mind focused on where you're going and what you want, not where you've been and what you don't want, and for that reason, we call them "Forward Focused." You'll use EQ's to get more positive, proactive, and productive thinking from yourself.

The solution to a problem lies in a completely different consciousness than the one that created the problem. You wouldn't have created your old reality in the first place had you been in a higher consciousness, but don't make yourself wrong—you're evolving.

> *EQ's help you reach that higher consciousness even when*
> *you don't have a clue how to get there.*

EQ's Are Open-Ended

EQ's stimulate the Infinity Factor, because the possibilities for how you can answer an open-ended question are endless. The awareness of unlimited possibilities frees you from Devil's Choices and limiting thinking.

ACTIVITY: Ask These EQ's Out Loud

Say them out loud and feel the shift as your vocal chords vibrate this way:

> *What miraculous possibilities exist that I don't yet know about?*
>
> *How might something come along that changes everything?*
>
> *What amazing things are headed my way?*
>
> *I wonder who or what can fill in these missing pieces?*
>
> *If some new miracle resource showed up, how would that feel?*

Bookstores rave about *Things Are Going Great*; it sells like hotcakes and people come back saying it's the best book they've ever read—but if bookstores don't know about it they can't order it. I wanted to buy a list of all metaphysical bookstores in the United States and mail them postcards about the book. But oddly, of all the databases you can buy, such a database did not exist, so I asked my assistant to find the stores on the Internet and *create* a database.

It was a task she really didn't want to undertake, so we asked this EQ as she went about other tasks: "*What's a better way to do this?*" Because of her resistance, it took a while, but she eventually found a man in the Philippines who would search out the addresses for her inexpensively, earning what for him is really good income.

Effective Questions activate your infinite creative power as they send your mind out on a productive hunting expedition unlimited by space or time. Your intention and some good EQ's can reach across the world to find just what you need.

*Effective Questions take you to a higher consciousness
or a completely new reality.*

You don't answer the EQ's; you ask them and let go. Your Larger Mind percolates on those EQ's even while you sleep, and will not stop until the best answer is found. It's like having your own creative staff waiting to go to work for you. I couldn't even list all the EQ's I've had answered— some fast, some more slowly. My part was to release resistance to believing it was possible.

Often, you find yourself in the middle of positive action, using the information or implementing the solution before you even realize it's the answer to an EQ you asked days or weeks before.

Ask, smile, and let go.

Intend and be receptive to the inspirations that come your way. Sometimes you don't have to do *anything* except ask; sometimes you must take the stepping-stones that lead you to it.

I promised you even more creative ways to "get out of the way" in this book. When you ask yourself EQ's, you send your mind on a mission. It's like giving the kids a fun puzzle to work so they'll stay out of the way while you get some work done, except with EQ's, your Larger Self gets the work done with your limiting mind out of the way.

Making flat statements can cause people, or your own mind, to resist you. People don't resist EQ's because EQ's don't *push; they pull* resourcefulness from people, bringing out their best. EQ's are one of my favorite ways to raise vibration or lure the mind away from problem-focus.

The mind often argues with affirmations, "Liar, liar, pants on fire. That's not true!" because affirmations fly directly in the face of current reality. EQ's don't contradict or demand, they're just innocent, uplifting questions.

EQ's are as irresistible to the mind as a feather on a string is to a cat. The mind is compelled to go after it.

*The Presence can help you most when
your mind is going with the flow.*

Practice asking forward-focused, open-ended EQ's instead of backwards-focused, yes/no, or scary questions. Don't work at it, just play with it, until it's a habit. The minute you think about creating a new possibility or solving a challenge, ask yourself things like these:

How satisfying will it be to have more ease?

How much fun can I make this? Can you feel the intention going into effect here? Just asking sets an intention, while releasing the tension of having to know the answer or do it right this minute.

How good will it feel when I have a new habit?

How do people who are successful in romantic relationships vibrate?

What will I do with my time when money is a non-issue?

EQ's can also begin with "where" or "who:"

Where could I connect with people who would love help?

Who are the people who are looking for me?

Where might I discover some helpful information?

Ask, SMILE, and let go.

If it's hard to let go, try out these EQ's:

How could I feel or see this completely differently?

What would help me relax and soften about this?

How can I feel better?

What would help get me out of the way?

How can I give this over to The Presence?

How can I adjust my attitude about this just a little?

Here's another variation that will soften even the most cynical of minds:

Wouldn't it be nice if . . . ? It's the intention and the feeling, not the form of the question that makes it an EQ.

What if I woke up tomorrow and felt completely different?

What would help even a little bit?

How could this get just a little bit easier day by day?

I wonder how I could open up to let in more?

What would (my role model) do?

Wouldn't it be cool if something I never thought of came along that's even better than what I lost?

Ask, SMILE, and let go.

* * * * * * * *

Closed-Ended Questions Are Dead-End Questions

- Close-ended questions are dead-ended because they can only be answered with a yes or no.
- They don't stimulate imagination or open up new possibilities.
- They don't send your mind on a helpful seek-and-find mission.
- They *feel* like an interrogation designed to place blame.

Can I do this? Did I do all I could?

Was it my fault? Did I do something wrong?

Am I not smart enough? Do I have the resources?

Can I do this without a degree? Will they like me?

Will I end up a failure?

There is no reality in the answers to those questions. You make it up. You make it true or not—with your belief and your emotional energy.

Ask Scary Questions—Get Scary Answers!

The mind loves to tell scary stories and ask scary questions. Scary questions multiply fear in the same way EQ's multiply wonderful new possibilities. Considering the hypnotic-command-power of EQ's, you wouldn't want to send your mind on a quest for scary things!

Scary Open-Ended Questions: Just because it starts with "what" or "how" doesn't make it an EQ.

What if I'm not smart/pretty/talented enough?

What if I can't do it?

What if I end up homeless?

How could this go wrong?

What if I lose my job?

What if she takes my husband?

What if someone takes advantage of me?

How stupid will I feel if I fail?

What if things never change for me?

What if the company fails and I have no retirement?

What if it is impossible and I'm in big trouble?

Ask scary questions—you get scary answers.

Doubt Your Doubts
Convert Scary Questions To EQ's

People often question their dreams and desires—and everyone considers that normal, wise, and even fair! Turn the tables. Ruthlessly question, challenge, and doubt your doubts!

Question your doubts and pick them apart; interrogate your fears and counter-intentions. Creative EQ's sneak up behind your limiting beliefs and knock the legs out from under them. Playfully put a fatal crack in the foundation, and the crack widens until it falls apart.

Doubt your doubts!

Sometimes it's better to be uncertain. Use Effective Questions to challenge *limiting certainties* and open new doors. Here we address the scary questions above, but we don't try to refute or resist them—we gently redirect your mind toward finding other possibilities:

What if... I just possibly AM smart enough?

What if... it isn't quite as hard as I thought?

What if... I DON'T end up homeless?

How could this maybe NOT go wrong?

I wonder… what if I DON'T lose my job?

What if my relationship turns out to give me a lifetime of happiness?

How could I make sure no one takes advantage of me?

What would happen if I didn't feel stupid?

I wonder… how could things change for me?

What if an even better situation comes along?

It's fun to wonder how other possibilities might appear?

How can I know what's possible or not in this amazing Universe?

How could I be so sure it won't all work out fabulously?

How could I have more fun discovering the solution to this?

What if this limitation isn't as cut and dried as I thought?

What if there are possibilities I haven't even imagined?

How could I absolutely positively KNOW there's no solution when possibilities are so vast and unlimited?

What if it ISN'T impossible?

How many times have I thought I'd exhausted all options, and there were more, like Thomas Edison's thousand attempts to invent a light bulb?

How can I know for sure it won't work when I haven't tried everything and the game is not over yet?

What if I was even slightly open to the possibility of a resolution?

How many stories are there in which something entirely unexpected and new shows up?

Question all scary questions.

Ask, SMILE, and let go.

* * * * * * * *

Backward Focus

"Backwards focus" keeps us fixated on the past or the problem and holds us out of vibrational range of the answers. When we're down in the valley with the problem, we can't see the solution at the top of the hill. If your ears are tuned to the problem frequency, you've got to shift to the radio station the wisdom is being broadcast on in order to hear it.

ACTIVITY: How Does It Feel?

Is the question useful? Soothing? Forward or backward focused? If it takes you deeper into limitation, backwards, or into the scary story, it's not helping you. Just for contrast, answer these questions and notice which way you go and how you feel:

Why did my parents fail me?

What is wrong with me?

Why is my lover not here yet?

Why is it so hard to get a job?

How could I have been so dumb?

Why can't I ever get out of debt?

Why am I sick?

Why am I so fearful?

It's okay to glance backward briefly, to get clear on what you don't want, but if you keep your head twisted around too long, you'll trip over something. Notice how when you're driving and you look at something off the road, you veer that way without meaning to. Watch where you point that thing.

You tend to go in the direction you're looking.

Why Ask Why?

"Why . . . ?" questions are usually not EQ's, even though they are open-ended. If you answer the questions below, the answers take you down the Instrument Panel. If any question drops your vibration, focuses you on what's wrong or doesn't forward-focus you toward new possibilities, it's not an EQ, even if it looks like one technically.

Why doesn't he love me?

Why do I have problems with my mother?

Why do things always go wrong?

Why do I always have more expenses just as I get ahead?

Why don't I improve?

Why me, God?

Why questions can help if only you use them as feedback to gain awareness, or to help you do it better next time:

Why did that happen?

Why didn't they hire me?

Or switch to actual EQ's:

What could I do better next time?

How could I communicate better?

What preparation do I need?

Who could coach me on making a better presentation?

Now, Have Fun With EQ's!

EQ's help you let go and let The Divine do the heavy lifting, offering you more ease, flexibility, creativity, and joy. Now it's time to get really creative with EQ's and have some fun. Delight yourself with inventive and ingenious ones that light you up just by asking them:

What would change the whole game rather than finding a better way to play the old game?

How can I add joy to this world?

Won't it be nice when the economy is thriving?

How might something better come along than what I'm set on?

What could I do differently?

What could I let go of?

How could it work out in a most unusual and delightful way?

How great will it be when…?

What could help that I don't currently know about?

Who might I serendipitously meet?

To get yourself in positive expectation and playful curiosity, ask:

> *What cool stuff will I experience when I'm more in the flow?*
>
> *How might it be different and better than I expected?*
>
> *How will these colors dance together in this painting?*
>
> *Won't it be fun when I get out of the way?*
>
> *How much fun will it be?*
>
> *How delighted will I be?*
>
> *What will I discover?*

Ask, SMILE, and let go.

These options have the same intention and effects of an EQ:

> *I wonder what would change the whole game for me?*
>
> *I wonder what great surprises are in store?*
>
> *Won't it be fun when . . . . ?*
>
> *Wouldn't it be great if . . . ?*
>
> *Wouldn't it blow my mind if . . . ?*

We can make up conscious questions that call forth our inner wisdom instead of seeking answers from other people. In the old paradigm, we'd ask someone, "Which is the correct next stepping-stone?" Later, we would laugh because that makes no sense in the new paradigm. In the new paradigm you "creatively wonder" about it and the right stepping-stone appears exactly when you need it.

Out on the leading edge, established answers are often not available. Imagine Lewis and Clark stopping to ask for a road map; Armstrong, Aldrin, and Collins looking for street signs on the way to the moon; Alexander Fleming, who accidentally discovered penicillin, looking in a textbook for the answer to the question, "What is this substance growing in my petri dish good for?"

Effective Questions support the theme of this book—that you can access the unlimited power of your Larger Non-Physical Being, calling upon its unlimited resources beyond our human capacity.

Humans are narrow-focused by design, which is good, because we deal with and create through the contrast and details of life, but a too-narrow focus eliminates options. EQ's deliberately cast a broad net and tap you into your Large Self's broader focus—a wonderful counterpoint.

The answer is always available.
Ask Effective Questions.

The Level Two Online Retreat includes many supporting audios and videos about EQ's and gives more examples of them.

EQ's Summary:

- EQ's are useful and helpful, whereas some questions are not.
- The mind doesn't resist EQ's. The mind doesn't argue with them like it often does with affirmations, demands, or commands.
- A statement confronts, a question invites.
- The mind gets caught up in answering the question (there are a million possible answers) and forgets to resist, doubt, or debate.
- They're only teasers, so they don't seem threatening. They don't demand you believe them, they only suggest.
- EQ's invite you to slip into a wonderful world of possibilities and curiosity.
- They don't ask that you do anything, just to consider some options, so resistance is further lowered.
- They invite you to expand your view without committing to anything.
- They allow you to relax while things get done in the Non-Physical.
- They ignore (rather than resist) the finite and focus on the Infinite.

ACTIVITY: Write EQ's that delight you and make you smile.

EQ's are useful in everything you do. Play with them often, talking to your Large Self until it's your natural habit to ask EQ's. Create some to fit your current desires and needs, or just for joy and expansion:

1.

2.

3.

4.

5.

6.

7.

Ask, SMILE, and let go.

* * * * * * * *

Counter-Intentions From The Collective

Limiting beliefs are all-too-easy to pick up in childhood, before we know better, then, without our noticing, they begin to operate in the background of our adult lives and can act as counter-intentions that dilute our desires.

As you become more conscious, you challenge any limiting beliefs you have or are offered. Each time you replace unconscious limitations with conscious choices, you lift the entire collective. Here are some limitations offered by the collective consciousness, along with some empowering alternatives:

Collective limitation:	Deliberate intention or EQ:
There's not enough for everyone.	What if there is plenty?
There are haves and have-nots.	Shifting one's vibration makes everything possible.
There is good/bad, right/wrong.	The Presence doesn't judge.
You must earn everything you get.	Grace provides generously.
Life is hard.	How can I let it be easier for me?
Life is risky.	There is no risk for an eternal being.
Outside forces control our fate.	Our vibration creates our results.
Human power is limited.	The Presence is unlimited.
Spiritual people are always smiling.	Bliss can't always be seen.

Oddly enough, a high percentage of spiritual people pulse a subtle, persistent unworthiness. I've seen people decide to "get spiritual," start trying to "be good," work on themselves as if they've suddenly discovered something's wrong with them, and actually go downhill, go broke, or begin struggling.

Let go of the vibration that you must earn worthiness—or anything. Unworthiness is a total mistake; it exists nowhere in nature or Creation except in the wrong-seeking, judging human mind. You are not judged like you judge yourself.

Breathe in worthiness—breathe out doubt.

You are already adored, and Divine Openings or being spiritual doesn't make you better. The Presence already adores you more than you'll probably ever let in. Divine Openings doesn't make you more worthy or blessed—it just helps you claim the worthiness that's already yours and let in the blessings being offered to you.

When you sign up for a certain path in life, you can accidentally pick up baggage that goes with it. Even if you think you already dropped all the baggage that came with being spiritual, intend to jettison any remnants of it right now. For example: "Spiritual and pure equals self-sacrificial and meek." "Rich equals evil and greedy." "Corporations equal evil and greedy. I must quit my corporate job to make a difference."

Let go of the *materialistic view* that money has any intrinsic vibration in and of itself. Let go of the belief that money or lack of money has anything to do with how good, bad, worthy, or unworthy you are. Let go of the belief that money has any power at all other than what you give to it.

Let go of worry that you can mess up, or that you can fail to measure up to the The Presence's standards or mission for you. You are perfect right now in the eyes of The Presence, and nothing further is required of you. Relax and enjoy life. Let go of any fear that you won't get what you want. Everyone gets it, whether in this lifetime or later ones. Intend to let it in now. It's your choice.

You're going to become even more powerful, so let go of any notions that power is bad. Intend to use it in a way that feels good.

Whoa, I Didn't Intend That!

"I didn't intend *that!*" someone might say. As you become more conscious, you notice how you are indeed attracting things inadvertently, like the man in prison suddenly becoming aware of how his insidious, invisible unworthiness had caused his downward spiral. Of course, he never said to The Presence or even to himself, "I am unworthy—take away all these good things I don't deserve, and ruin my life." He wasn't aware of his feelings of unworthiness until our session, which you can hear (with his voice and identity edited out) if you ever take Level Three Online—Jumping The Matrix.

There's a wonderful audio you can purchase separately and download at DivineOpenings.com called *How Did I Create THAT?* It's very soothing, and sheds light on how we create things unconsciously, for example, by having blind spots and counter-intentions.

If you're not fully conscious of what you're intending, you create a matrix of what you want, then another matrix of what you fear or don't want, and the two can split your energy. I've seen people vibrate themselves right into poverty when they try to prove to a spouse who's divorcing them that they cannot afford a divorce settlement. They want to avoid giving money by insisting that they don't have it, so the Universe says, "OK, you're right, you don't have money." That's also an advanced case of needing to be right and make the spouse wrong.

One friend had set the intention to get her finances in ship shape and pay off debt and was mystified why it wasn't happening. Her able-bodied and sweet but money-allergic sixty-five-year-old boyfriend had let her support him for their entire five years together, and she didn't value herself enough to stop enabling him, so she told tried complaining, "I can't afford to support you anymore." I asked her if she'd noticed that her dominant intention was to be *too poor to be able to support him,* and that her intention was coming true. I suggested saying to him truthfully, "I don't wish to support you anymore," while raving to her Large Self about her improving finances.

There are infinite varieties of hidden intention. Just intend to see it. What you're vibrating is right there for all to see. Others can often see it more clearly than you do.

A sure way to know what you're truly intending is to look at your life. Really. I don't mean how much material stuff you have, although that is certainly a nice little reflection of your money vibration. I mean the important stuff:

- Love—vibrationally matched relationships with family, lovers, and friends.
- Joy and fun.
- Satisfaction and passion you feel in your activities and work.
- How comfortable your home is, not necessarily how large or expensive.
- Health—how vital and relaxed your body is most of the time.
- What you bring out in those around you.
- The things that occur with, for, and to you.
- Daily experiences and interactions.
- Having enough money to meet your needs and bills, or more.
- How much you appreciate—or complain, and how that is reflected back to you.
- How you feel overall.
- How you feel in each department of your life.

Have a look. It's illuminating. Celebrate anywhere you can—tweak your intentions. Don't take score—use it as feedback, ask some EQ's, and get out of the way.

Your life is your intentions made visible.

Another aspect of human nature comes into play with some of the puzzling things we think we didn't intend. Humans really do love contrast and variety, although we may say we want only sweetness and light, goodness and bliss. Notice how you're drawn to look at an auto accident or read a news story with a shockingly perverse headline. The contrast of dark makes the light seem brighter. Being ill makes feeling good so much better. The longing for something you don't have makes it so much sweeter when it comes.

Intend to enjoy and even create contrast rather than falling into contrast by accident. You want the contrast of excitement in forms you choose, but not sticky drama that burdens you. Life will give you drama to wake you up if you don't do it yourself. As you become more conscious and develop your power of intention, you will choose expansion more deliberately, and get it less by pain and default.

A woman had an astrology reading, and the astrology chart said she'd soon face serious addiction problems. She believed astrology had power over her, so she made a conscious decision to play that drama out rather than become a victim of it. She took a role as Judy Garland in a theater production and exuberantly expressed the drama in that healthy way. Of course, she also could have refused to give the reading any power—I give astrology no power over me and don't even care to know about it—but she solved it from where she was, and enjoyed the pleasure of acting to boot!

There are Divine Openings Givers who have so little drama and contrast in their lives that they read dramatic novels. We joke that now that we don't have enough of that in our real lives so we get it vicariously from stories.

Your neurology is wired for contrast. You would not know what cold is if you didn't have heat. Heat is more precious to an Eskimo than to a resident of the tropics.

We all have a need for drama and contrast, dark and light, tears and laughter, up and down, challenge and relief, work and rest. When you're conscious of that, and you intentionally choose creative ways to play out those needs, you don't have to fall into drama unconsciously to get those needs met. You can take action with both eyes on your Instrument Panel, or you can default to falling backwards into what you're attracting vibrationally through unconscious intentions, and risk it coming in a form you don't really want. People blow up relationships simply looking for some excitement.

If you have a higher need for stimulation or adventure than most others, you'll need to challenge yourself even more. You respond well to big risks and may even dive into adrenaline sports or take on nearly impossible tasks. You like high tension and finding the relief from it; then you want to do it again. Things you find highly satisfying might be tortuous for a more contented, easy-going person.

Find your own balance of challenge and comfort.

Most people's taste for and experience of drama shrinks after doing Divine Openings, but if you have a higher need for stimulation, excitement, and contrast, find productive, non-destructive ways to feed that need.

One client is a rock star who dresses in astoundingly creative costumes and makeup, writes, performs, and makes videos of his completely unique music, yet when he initially called me, his mind was out of control and torturing him with scary stories that were coming true. He would achieve some success, then crash it dramatically, and go down in flames. He had a huge fear that the pattern would repeat itself, which of course it did.

After listening to him for a while, I said, "Your prolifically creative mind has a great appetite for drama, and your mind is always busily creating it. The untrained mind is a wrong-seeking missile—a fear generating, survival-obsessed machine. First of all, you must make a powerful decision that *your mind is not you* and you don't have to listen to everything it says. You don't have to follow where it leads and it is not allowed to be your master."

The untrained mind is a wrong-seeking missile.

Then I asked, "Second, how juicy, and gooey, and detailed do you make the scary stories? How much feeling, Technicolor, scary music in Dolby soundtrack, and action horror do you put in them? And, by contrast, how much do you dramatize your positive thoughts, hopes, and dreams? Do you put that much intention, and power, and drama into your hopeful stories, thoughts, and feelings?"

I quickly added, "Don't worry if the answer is no. You're not the only human who dramatizes the holy hell out of the scary stuff, and barely puts any intentional juice at all into dramatizing the stuff you want. Notice that the media does that, too—playing up the scary, negative drama and making the good stuff bland and wimpy. Humanity is so hooked on drama it might as well be crack cocaine. It does make you feel alive all right, but there are far more pleasant ways to feel fully alive."

"Your play for the next few weeks is to deliberately take charge of your mind, dramatize the *positive* aspects of your life and fill your need for high-drama that way. Fill your mind with productive drama, leaving less room for mischief. Go to the mirror and tell yourself your scary story, and see it for what it is. Then make up a juicy and dramatic story that ends happily."

The mind is an excellent servant, but a horrific master.

This and hundreds of other session recordings can be heard or downloaded from the self-paced online courses. People often say it doesn't always matter so much what the topic of the audio is— they'll just choose randomly or pick what calls to them and it applies to their need or desire. They often say it felt like I was speaking directly *to them*--interesting, because *my intention* with every audio is for it to speak to everyone who listens, not just the person being counseled.

Sometimes, I'll find myself in some mild drama, or displeased with some bad service, and I'll laugh that I must have needed some excitement or hadn't been giving myself enough adventure, challenge, and variety. As soon as I realize that I created it, I stop making it wrong—I might as well enjoy it once I've created it!

Any significant drama, especially getting sideways with a loved one, actually gives me a kind of hangover the next day. It hurts, and it's supposed to hurt when we drop down on the Instrument Panel. To me, it feels like an octopus-like creature is suction-cupped to my face. It's a navigational message, "Get back up there with your Large Self! It feels awful down here!"

When there's an alien on your face (vibration is low),
try to postpone critical conversations, actions, and decisions.

Know yourself, and be proactive in meeting your needs. Intend now to know yourself better and better, and make your intentions conscious. If you need excitement, you can create it deliberately rather than backing unconsciously into drama to meet that need. When you create more deliberately, you have fewer of those *"How did I create THAT?"* moments.

I create challenging new projects because I must create new things all the time. Maintaining the status quo is not enough for me, where others might just kick back and retire. That would be boring to me.

When I'm done, I'll depart the planet consciously. That's truly possible with some mastery of intention, and many people have accomplished conscious and deliberate dying. I would aspire to do it even if there was no evidence it could be done. I'd ask the EQ, "How can I consciously depart this body when I'm finished with it?"

Deepak Chopra tells a story about his father, who was a physician in India in his eighties when he arrived home one day after a full day of work and announced to his wife that he was "going." He lay down on the bed and entered "the big meditation" and left his body permanently. Maharishi, the founder of Transcendental Meditation, who found great fame when The Beatles studied with him, also left his body consciously. He sat on his lecture platform; devotees covered him and the platform with flowers, leaving only his face exposed, and he departed peacefully. That's an example of your will and God's will being one. People say only The Creator knows when we will depart, but that's only true if we are not in alignment with Source. There's no right or wrong way to transition, I just think it would be fun to do it consciously.

There are infinite applications for power of intention.

* * * * * * * *

Powerful Intention, Or Wishful Thinking?

Because you're making it all up—you make things true for you. Whether it's "true or not" isn't a useful distinction between a powerful intention and wishful thinking. Here's the distinction:

- Wishful thinking occurs when you're expecting something to happen but you're vibrating something contradictory to it.
- Or when you want something and you say you're creating it, but your vibration says you're not, and you're not doing anything to change how you're feeling or vibrating.

Example: two separate persons in different cities say, "I'm going to start a large alternative hospital." The first person is vibrating very powerfully in alignment with her desire, has cleaned up her counter-intentions, and is fully prepared to follow through all the way, doing the mundane, unglamorous details it will take to pull it off. She's willing to go on the ride even though she will need a lot of help and doesn't have all the answers. She's vibrationally lined up with her own intention enough to take steady, practical, successful steps, and she grows in the process. This is not wishful thinking at all—it's a powerful intention.

The second person's words and her vibration are not lined up. She doesn't read her Instrument Panel very well, so she can't feel counter-intentions splitting her energy. She expects her intention to show up even though her energy and her current stage of evolution don't match it. She is not prepared to focus and follow through with the daily details—she's more excited by the glamorous idea of it than the real day-to-day work. She likes the vision but isn't prepared to go on the journey. She wants it without having to change, stretch, and grow. This is wishful thinking.

The Overnight Millionaire

Overnight wealth can and does happen, but when people come to me wild-eyed after attending a How To Be A Millionaire Overnight seminar, and they're not feeling their feelings, can't read their Instrument Panel, don't understand how they've created the money shortage they're in now, and think wealth that doesn't match their current vibration is going to suddenly descend upon them, I suggest they slow down and focus on how they feel first.

Skip to the payoff, and feel better about money first.

If you want more money, start appreciating the life you have now, even small amounts of money or any loans you've been given. Do you realize that loans are someone *giving you money* merely on your promise to pay them back with interest? That is a miraculous manifestation. Appreciate that *right now.*

Focus only on how you're feeling, and pay attention to your Instrument Panel. Reach for, intend, and nurture the feeling you think money will bring you—cultivate it *now.* Once you do that, you know precisely and clearly where you stand in your ability to let in a certain amount of money. You can feel if you're pulsing, "I let money in," or not.

If it makes you more aware of the lack of money, then don't affirm, "I'm a millionaire." It just frustrates you and throws you out of integrity because it's contradictory to what you're vibrating. You can say those words later, once you're vibrating closer to them.

Build small successes at first and let your evidence and belief escalate. Better to speak something you can actually feel, such as, "Little bits of money are coming to me more and more easily all the time," and begin to stack up some evidence. In a few months or a year, you'll end up believing yourself when you say, "Money is a non-issue in my world." Start where you are.

My Tennessee-born mom looks at a plate piled with more food than the person can eat and says, "Your eyes are bigger than your stomach." Translating this to the Divine Openings context, "Your desires are higher than your vibration." There is nothing more frustrating! Go back to minding how you're feeling and what you're pulsing—you can do something about that right now, while you can't change your financial or health condition right this minute. Let go, enjoy life, and take incremental steps every day toward your desires.

Thinking, "The Universe will give it to me if I intend to share it and not be selfish," doesn't work. Being "good" doesn't get you anything—the Universe doesn't care if you're selfish or unselfish with money—it just responds to your vibration. Bribing God isn't an option! Gangsters get money because they believe they can; they only get arrested when they vibrate guilt. Being good doesn't get you anything—vibrating high on a topic does.

If someone tells me he wants to win the lottery, I'll ask him if he's vibrating in alignment with that possibility. If he's not really feeling it, I suggest he pick something that's less of a stretch that he can believe. Curiously, this can open the door to bigger boons faster because there's less resistance.

I'd rather see my reality expand every year *in response to my increasing power of intention* rather than give the lottery even the tiniest bit of power over my fate. The lottery is not the source of my happiness, freedom, or money—Source is the source of that, and can deliver it to all of us in the perfect way. One person in millions can win the lottery, yet all of us can create financial ease and have all the good feelings we think the lottery would give us if we commit to learning how:

> Decide on the feelings you want about money, skip to the payoff, and start enjoying those very feelings right now. The high vibrational signal you pulse forms a Non-Physical matrix (template, blueprint, outline, general plan) of your new creation. Using the unlimited resources of the Universe, your Non-Physical Self, fills in the material forms best for you. It is not even your job to know how to flesh it out—your job is to create the skeletal matrix by intention, and go with the flow.

Thinking, "More money will solve all my problems and make me happy," gives too much power to the material world. Vibrate higher and higher on a topic and watch the outside world line up with that.

When you create it, it means something.

If you pay attention primarily to how you feel rather than to what material things you're popping into the physical, you'll pay more attention to what really matters: your vibration and your alignment with the Non-Physical.

People often ask me why I don't do this or that big, ambitious thing with Divine Openings, like be on television or give more events. Answer: I'm very much enjoying the steady, incremental rise of Divine Openings and living a sane, integrated life, not chasing after anything. In this steady, step-by-step way, I adapt to the growth at each new level, and never slip back.

I truly never imagined being where I am now, and if I'd been thrown into this too quickly, it would have been hard to let it all in at once. When a boon is "beyond belief," literally beyond one's ability to let it be real, it can be hard to maintain it.

It's not about having it all right now—
it's about enjoying each new expansion.

* * * * * * * *

The Pleasure And Power Of Silence

Miriam, a participant in a Five Day Silent Retreat, went very deep into the powerful silence. She was camping at a nearby park during the retreat, and as she was walking to the bathhouse one day, she passed with a woman with a gorgeous dog. Miriam didn't want to break her silence, and was practicing saying everything to The Presence, so she formed the words in her mind, "What a beautiful dog." The woman said, "Thank you." Miriam's intention was so powerful the woman heard it without words! Stay still and quiet inside as much as you can.

Scientists are looking for rational, logical explanations of how creatures like whales and dolphins communicate, and when they discover them, they will probably be as simple as "by intention," but that may not be complicated or physical enough to satisfy science.

Notice how much you talk. Usually, the more you talk, the less you say, and the more your power of intention drains. Notice if you feel compelled to talk and can't stop talking whether people are listening or not.

Some people talk to avoid feeling, using their words like an anesthetic or drug—like an addiction—to drown themselves in floods of unnecessary words. When a client does that, I ask her to stop talking and just feel. She calms down and gets better. If I let her keep gushing, nothing changes because she's avoiding the feeling by talking.

Begin to cultivate more silence with those you love. People listen more as you talk less. You don't have to talk to commune deeply, as people discover in the Five Day Silent Retreat. Sit, enjoy, feel, and savor together.

You can increasingly relate with others for pure love and enjoyment rather than need. Play replaces commiseration and problem-solving. Joy and connection replace disconnection and "relationship issues." If there is something uncomfortable between you, take your intention for the relationship to The Presence first and get clear on your intention. If your intention is to get the other person to change or admit she's wrong, you'll recognize that in the clarity of silence, and find a larger intention.

Dive in privately first, with the intention to clean up your own vibration and feel the other person's point of view objectively. Once you feel calm and powerful, speak from the heart to the other person.

As you talk less, keep your own counsel, and enjoy the blessed silence more, your power of intention grows—just one more example of how this book is more about what you *don't do* than what you *do*—what you *let go* of more than what you *add*.

For about six weeks, or until it becomes a habit, talk to The Presence within more than you speak out loud. The potency of your words and intentions exponentially increase as you dilute them less with "filler" words and intentions. As you speak to, ask for advice from, and rely on The Presence rather than other people, your Oneness with The Presence deepens.

Keep your own counsel to build inner power.

Fold The Good Back In

When we talk too much, energy is scattered verbally. When we communicate internally with The Presence we don't scatter or leak energy, we compound it, as if we've put our money in a bank and earned interest on it instead of spending it on trinkets. I call this *folding the energy back in*. When we *do* choose to speak, we're spending that verbal energy wisely, consciously, and more gets accomplished with that energy.

In the Five Day Silent Retreat, people are astounded to find out just how much energy they have been using by speaking. Speaking is a left-brain activity that activates the mind. Not speaking quiets the mind. After going deep in the Five Day Retreat, some of us are in no rush to leave the sheer ecstasy of the silence. Small talk is actually painful to me after those retreats.

If you feel like you must speak to someone, notice why you really need it. Do you need love, attention, sharing? Do you want admiration, approval, validation, support, or soothing? Feel the desire to talk, and instead of talking, dive into the feeling with The Presence. When you take your joys and your challenges within, you get over outer dependence and discover the real power you can't get from other people.

Intend to make it *enough* to share it inside. Big things happen when the Non-Physical becomes more important and real to you than the physical.

Take your joy and your challenges inside
rather than scattering energy outside.

Humans do seem to need an awful *lot* of validation from others, and those who let go of that become truly *free*. Particularly those who choose to live on the leading-edge cannot count on mainstream validation, or even validation from spiritual friends. If I were the only person on the planet who lives the way I do, it wouldn't concern me at all. Over my lifetime the "weird" things I've always done have eventually become accepted, but at first they were rejected as being too new, unproven, or different from the mainstream.

People ask how to know yourself as The Presence—not just in theory, but in practice. It's the same as building any important intimate relationship: give it quality time, and prioritize it. Spend time with The Presence in silence. Fold your joy back in. Reinvest it.

Make it <u>enough</u> to say it to yourself and The Presence.

Summarizing, to compound your power of intention:

- Spend time in deep silence with no words or thoughts.
- Talk to The Presence more than other people.
- Fold it back in, compound the good feelings like interest rather than "spending" or scattering them.

ACTIVITY: Take It All Within.
Take some weeks to point *virtually all* of your communication inside, speaking to yourself as The Presence, instead of pointing outward at other people. This is what I did for a solid twenty-one days some years ago, and my power of intention increased exponentially. If there are other people you must talk to, make your words as concise and powerful as you can. Life gets better and better when you watch where you point that thing.

* * * * * * * *

How Much Action Is Required?

How much blood, sweat and tears does it take to have things happen? How much physical effort does it take to get things done, make a living, or build a dream?

When I talk about Ease and Grace that doesn't mean I don't have to do anything. Grace does do ninety percent of it for us when we get out of the way, and ninety-nine percent of all manifestation does happen on the Non-Physical level before it begins to materialize in the physical, so things can be accomplished easier than most people believe possible. By letting Grace do more for us, and by putting more of our attention and focus on how we're creating (or un-creating) in the Non-Physical, we can, as I've said, *cut our action to a fraction.*

When your pipes are open and you can let it in, Grace leads you to the easiest and best options possible, and causes lesser options to fall through.

On the Non-Physical level, you get the energy lined up before toiling in the denser physical world. It's easier because once you've assembled the energy template or matrix of any "thing" or experience, the manifestation is already mostly complete. Sometimes people waffle at that stage, getting it almost complete, then doubting it and delaying it; getting it almost complete, then reversing it by feeling bad about it; getting it almost complete, then remembering how it didn't happen in the past.

Get in alignment with your Large Self on the chosen intention, let go of all the roadblocks (resistances and counter-intentions) you've thrown up in front of yourself; know it's coming even when you don't see it yet, and keep skipping to the payoff. That's called staying out of the way.

Your job is to feel good.

That last bit of a creation is physical, however, and someone (that's you and me) has to draw up the plans, raise the funds, hire the people, and maybe even stack bricks and mortar ourselves. Maybe you need to apply for an entry-level job in the field you want to enter, paint your picture and ask to display it, or let people know what you can offer them. Spiritual people may have to get over biases and judgments about money, or "marketing," which essentially means "letting people know how you can help them."

You came here to do things, get your hands dirty, stretch your mind and your muscles, scrape your knuckles, stub your toe, and shape the clay of the physical world. If you'd wanted to float in ecstasy all the time, you'd have stayed in the Non-Physical.

You wanted expansion and adventure.

When you're clear what you really want, and you're willing to do what it takes to be, do, or have it, stay alert for the signs, cues, and openings to act. Act when urges strike, even though you don't have all the pieces. Be willing to be led without having all the answers or a clearly marked path.

Take baby steps and stay flexible. Don't nail it down until you get that solid feeling that says "yes." Things change quickly in this era. A graduate of the Five Day Silent Retreat told me the website she built five months ago now feels out of date. I can relate—I update mine almost daily because everything is evolving so fast.

The balance between physical and Non-Physical is not a one-time adjustment after which you're done forever. Like a good tightrope walker, you make constant adjustments. Sometimes people keep seeking, trying to find a way to create something with no physical effort, when they'd be better off taking some mundane physical steps. Children learn to walk by trying and falling down, not by thinking about it, planning, and waiting for a magical key. Of course, intention plays a part. Their strong desire for the freedom and independence of walking inspires them to keep practicing until they get it. There is a matrix for walking inside every child, and bit-by-bit, they grow into it physically.

Rather than waiting for something huge to fall in your lap, intend, which creates a corresponding matrix; then take small and steady physical steps as The Presence guides you to fill in the physical aspects of your new matrix.

Take a course in your desired area of accomplishment, whether it's computers, business management, law, real estate, art, or singing. If you want your business to do better, learn to market yourself, network more, or work on your offerings to make them more accessible, irresistible, beneficial, or useful in the marketplace.

Bring joy to the doing of it.

Some of us benefit from studying how successful people did it. Personally, I often do things completely differently than most people do them, and that works for me. I do take advice from those who have succeeded before me when it comes to technical solutions, because that is their genius and their area of focus, but not mine.

To take certain roads and ignore others requires a strong pull from within, not an intellectual decision. For example, no matter how much people tell me social media is the wave to ride, I don't enjoy it at all, so I've automated my Facebook and Twitter inspirational communications.

Does it feel good to me?

Toil And Struggle vs. Healthy Work And Challenge

I like to reframe the whole concept of work. Sometimes people think they don't want to have to work anymore, and I think that's just due to the oppressive way they're currently creating their work. Work is wonderful. I love work. If you stop challenging and pushing your physical body's muscles, they can weaken and atrophy, and you risk aging prematurely. But when you sweat and push yourself—walk, lift weights, do yoga or sports—your muscles strengthen and grow, and you stay young and healthy. Work offers that stimulation for your mind and spirit.

You know what happens to a lot of people who retire and have no reason to stay vital—they withdraw their life force from their body and exit the physical plane. Go for expansion, challenge, and a bit of exertion in this life to keep yourself alive and vital and growing. Now, pushing rocks up hills and toiling in the salt mines are not the kind of challenges we recommend. But hey, if you enjoy that kind of thing, do it!

At my age, fifty-eight at the time of this writing, it's particularly important to me not to stagnate in any way—body, mind, or spirit—but I will never again toil or struggle. I'm always challenging myself, expanding my "work" and beginning something new that I don't know how to do.

The many-months-long process of selling one home, packing, buying another home, and moving across the country stretched and expanded me. It was a lot of work, beginning with paring down the amount of stuff in the old house to stage it more attractively for showing, repairing things I had let slide, and going through the emotional journey of letting go of a place filled with happy memories. Then, there was the travel back and forth for the simultaneous selling and buying of homes.

Because of the mortgage-banking meltdown, the route to purchasing a home had radically changed since I bought my ranch ten years before, so I went from feeling like an experienced buyer to being an amateur. Each day, I learned new things about the new rules of mortgages, and each step brought new understanding of how to align with my Large Self on the Non-Physical to allow flow in the physical. It brought new awareness of thoughts and attachments that needed to evolve.

Physical life was so distracting for a while there—I fell out of my usual habit of staying in the stillness at the eye of the hurricane and got whipped out into the swirling chaos of my self-created cyclone a few times. Everything's relative, so my experience wasn't bad by most standards—it was just less wonderful than usual. Once you're accustomed to flying high, even a small drop in altitude feels really bad. It's *supposed to feel bad* so you want to get back up there.

Each time I got stuck, I'd endeavor to get out of the way, and each time I got out of the way, new possibilities arose. At one point, when I felt particularly in the flow, the lending rules changed overnight, allowing a dramatic reduction in the amount of down payment I had to pay, which meant I qualified for a much better house, with cash from the other sale left over to fix it up.

Each time something fell through or was delayed, I chose to celebrate—appreciating that Life had other plans lined up for me. Two homes I liked all right fell through, which made me nervous, because my Texas home had already gone under contract and I would soon need to depart. Russell and I would have to move our two households and two horses twice if something didn't show up soon.

That delay allowed time for the wonderful home we now live in to become available—my realtor heard about it before it the day before it was to go on the market—no other potential buyers were aware of it yet. This house and its location were the first that actually met all our needs without compromising. We were able to close on it right after my Austin home closed. I enjoyed being "homeless" for ten days while the furniture and horses made their way to California.

This World Of Contrasts

You and The Creator are capable of creating with intention alone, but you came here expressly to have physical experiences, go through physical processes, and experience unfolding in space/time. The eternal Non-Physical aspect of you that creates purely by intention comes here to have contrasting experiences that you can't have when you're all-knowing, all-seeing, timeless, Non-Physical, and able to manifest anything instantly with a mere thought.

In the Non-Physical, your state is steady, always blissful and "heaven-like". But in the physical, there is distance and separation, objects have mass, and things occur in timelines, or so it appears.

In the physical, you experience variety, polarity, and contrasts: hot/cold, up/down, slow/fast, light/dark, hard/soft, having/lacking, ecstasy/despair. You repeatedly and eagerly project aspects of yourself to play with these opposites and contrasts that don't exist in the Non-Physical.

Contrast does not mean "bad" or "things you don't like." It means simply that there is a wide range of experiences and choices, and you're bound to like some more than others.

You could have kept all of your Beingness in the Non-Physical if you'd wanted to. But you didn't. You signed up to experience this physical life and many other dimensions simultaneously, but this is the one we're concerned about right now. You chose this, with all its challenges, joys, and variety.

You may judge some human acts as disastrous, but in the Larger scheme of life, your Large Self loves experience for the sake of experience. You could say The Presence is an experience junkie, a glutton for adventure. And of course, from the Non-Physical, eternal perspective, it's all just experience, and there's never a failure or an end, just more, and more, and more.

Divine Openings brings Grace and ease, but you never wanted it *all* to be done for you. If you prevented a child from learning to walk or do anything on his own, carrying him around all the time trying to help him avoid failure, you'd cripple that child for life.

You wanted to use your Free Will to make choices, to act on and shape your environment, and have physical experiences that mirror your choices back to you. You wanted to feel your way, reading your Instrument Panel, celebrating your successes or correcting your course.

Hey, anybody can be happy when everything is always perfect—there's no mastery in that. You wanted to exercise your power out on this frontier, not just have everything handed to you ready made. You get to *exercise* your mastery, moving toward what you want and bouncing off things you don't want—deliberately using your power of intention, and honing your choices. "Oh, that isn't quite it, well I'll try this." And those bounces often take you somewhere you'd otherwise never have thought to go.

In 1856, William Perkins was trying to invent artificial quinine to cure malaria, but his experiment yielded a gooey mauve-colored substance. Fortunately, however, he noticed the beautiful color, and his curiosity led him to try it as a dye. His dye was superior to natural dyes, brighter, and non-fading. Science became a moneymaking endeavor for the first time just as Perkins was beginning to find practical life applications for his discoveries, leading many gifted people like him to make science their career. They created a new flood of inventions that forwarded evolution. One of the many people inspired by Perkin's work was a German bacteriologist, Paul Ehrlich, who used Perkin's dyes to pioneer immunology and chemotherapy.

Bounce off things you don't want.

There's value and purpose in the time things can take to create. You chose not to have every single thing work out instantly. You chose an unfolding experience with trial and error, choosing and re-choosing, creating and refining your creations. You may think you want all ease and no challenge or contrast, but you had that in the Non-Physical and you deliberately created a physical aspect of yourself here.

Humans love to play in the physical world. Athletes want to run a faster mile, and they are willing to push their bodies and work extremely hard to do it. Scientists seek better fuels and materials. Chefs strive to cook a more delicious dish, and they can stand the heat and pressure in the kitchen to do it. Dog whisperers get canines to do remarkable things no one thought they could do. Computer designers race to make ever smaller, faster, more powerful computers.

Ideally they enjoy the experience of it, not just the outcome. Those who wish simply to be done are missing out on the joy of life. Choose something you love to do, and feel the life force flowing through you as you do it. Enjoy the passing of time. Enjoy the sun on your face and the sweat on your brow.

Can you imagine The Creator lamenting, "When am I going to be finished with this creation? It's been going on forever and ever and still I'm not done. I can't wait to retire and play a little golf!" That's ridiculous, right? The primary imperative for The Creator is to expand, experience, and create endlessly. There is no expectation of a single outcome, or an end. It's not about that.

You came here intending to create a balance
of challenge and ease.

* * * * * * * *

Guidance Plus Life Experience

When you're not resisting, wild horses can't hold you back. You take action with joyful expectation, knowing that the way was laid out for you when you created your matrix of intention—but it's up to you to begin, walk down the paths, and choose the forks to take.

Watch the film *The Butcher's Wife* with the idea of following guidance in mind. Marina, our protagonist, was born a psychic, but even the most intuitive human's interpretations sometimes get distorted or clouded in the thick of this messy and distracting life. Due to the overriding goodness of life, even her erroneous assumptions result in entertaining misadventures that work out in the end. She quite accurately tells other people what she sees for them, but they also must interpret her words, find *their* way, and take their own steps and risks to finally discover where Life is leading them.

In the end you see how the matrices of everyone's desires fill in perfectly, despite apparent missteps along the way. If Marina hadn't made her initial, pivotal "mistake," Eugene wouldn't have become a famous artist, the gay couple would never have gotten together, Stella wouldn't have met her ideal man, the butcher might have remained single his whole life, and Marina might never have met her own true love. Although it plays out very differently than any of them imagined it would, the pieces all fall into place as everyone finds the flow.

Your guidance just might lead you through one expansion, then another and another, until finally you're ready to be led to "the place," "the person," or the experience your heart desires.

The route may be a winding river that flows southward to the sea—yet due to hairpin turns it's sometimes going north instead of south—seemingly the opposite direction of its destination. Or it might quickly lead you directly to the sea—one day I pondered, "Should I take vitamin D to help prevent aging?" and the next day saw a definitive cutting-edge article that answered yes.

The concept of Facebook did not come to its inventor fully formed—far from it. He started out by hacking into Ivy League college directories to find photos to help create a game that rated how pretty girls at the school were. (The Presence doesn't judge worthiness, merit, or morality.) His idea was wildly popular, and attracted investors who wanted an exclusive online directory for their club members. From there, he split off and began to develop Facebook. Once he got the company launched, he undertook extensive training and executive coaching to get himself up to speed with a role he was otherwise quite unprepared for.

Instant manifestation isn't the point—
the expansion you go through is of the greatest value.

Choose

As you read this book, your consciousness expands, so I repeat key elements in many different ways, because everyone hears it in some ways better than others. When you read it again, you'll get more.

Choose to stay focused on:

- Your inner reality, your Larger reality, rather than temporary physical reality.
- Large Self perspective. Closing your eyes, breathing softly, and asking this EQ instantly and completely shifts perception: *"How does my Large Self experience this?"*
- How you want to feel. Skip to the payoff.
- What you wish to experience, not whatever temporary thing is distracting you at the moment.
- The stillness within, where all is well, always.

Everything on the physical plane is temporary.

Of course, you and I are the creators of it all, but when we lose sight of that temporarily, it can feel like it's happening "to us." It's all part of the game of Life—this wonderfully expansive game of staying conscious and awake.

When you win this game, your prize is a great life. This game never ends, so there's never a final score. It's a fun game, but there's never a day when you can get lazy and stop choosing. I can't afford to get sloppy any more than you can. With the gift of Free Will comes the responsibility to keep choosing.

Practice "Devotion To Awakeness," the strong commitment to stay in your power.

Re-commit and re-devote yourself to Your Self. I don't mean *work* at it; intend and choose daily. Failing to choose is also a choice.

Yes, due to your ability to make Free Will choices, it is possible to lose your enlightenment, just as it is possible to go to sleep at the wheel of your vehicle and run off the road, no matter how alert you were twenty minutes ago.

It can be tempting to say, "Well, the economy is bad, so that's why my finances aren't improving," or "I can complain about my co-workers, because it's their fault," or "My spouse is the problem," but it costs us. It's just not worth it.

Stay awake. Catch yourself, and refocus.

- What do I want? Intend it powerfully, stubbornly.
- How would I like it to be? Skip to the payoff.
- How quickly can I get myself to say, "I created that"?
- How can I reclaim my power? Get into your Large Self.

You'll feel better instantly and move on.

I suppose I could simply sit back and do very little at this point in my life, but a bird flies and sings because it's a bird. That bird doesn't ever quit singing. My work moves energy through me, keeping me stimulated and happy. The Presence doesn't judge or demand that we fulfill some mission—that is New Age bunk or a distorted mistranslation of guidance.

Sometimes people think they want a kind of permanent vacation, which I think would actually be a type of walking death. Stagnation is not the kind of ease I want. Engage in life! Generate excitement and stimulation.

On Doing Practices

Some spiritual paths involve doing practices and working on yourself throughout your life. Oh, dear, that's boring, plus the very act of constantly affirming that you're not there yet keeps you from ever *being there*. Divine Openings lets you *be there now*. You expand constantly through these remarkable Divine Openings automatic downloads, with no need to work on yourself or "process." Life "processes you," if you will—desire, contrast, and the incoming evolutionary energies provide more than enough impetus to expand and evolve—all you do is let go and go with it. Practices give way to *intending* and *allowing* ongoing evolution.

As I explain in *Things Are Going Great In My Absence*, the formal practice of Diving In was created only to get you back into the natural habit of feeling in the moment—restoring you to the natural way of being that was trained out of you early in life. If I'm in huge resistance, I will do a Divine Openings practice or process, but as long as I'm in the flow of life there's no need to do anything but live, respond, enjoy, and evolve.

Just before you go to sleep and as your first undertaking when you wake, focus on what you appreciate, how you wish to feel that day, soar on a good feeling, and give yourself a high start for the day ahead. That's not work, that's pleasure.

Take charge if that wrong-seeking missile of a mind greets you in the morning with everything that's screwed up, needs solving, or is weighing on you.

Prostrating can help give your body/mind a powerful "let go" signal. It's explained in detail in *Things Are Going Great In My Absence*.

Life is simple. Only the mind makes it complicated.

Once your mind is tuned to good habits, negative thoughts occur less often. But again, you will never stop experiencing the negative contrasts that urge you on to higher evolution, and your mind will never stop looking for what could go wrong—it thinks it's protecting you. Find a balance in which you appreciate contrasts giving you something to bounce off of, but don't let contrasts make you suffer—just use them as juice to help you move.

One practice you might continue is meditation with the intention of pleasure, just because it feels so good. Yet if it ever becomes "work," its effectiveness and power will diminish.

Visit The Fertile Void

The Fertile Void is a place that is not even a place. Like The Presence, it's non-manifest—it's Nothing. It's beyond time and space and beyond definition, so keep in mind that no matter how you try to visualize it or figure it out, you can't.

You could think of it as the dark, velvety womb of Creation. There's nothing there, yet all potential resides there. There's nothing there, yet everything comes from there and returns to there. It's pre-manifest, pre-materialization, but all manifestations spring from it, from Nothing.

When we focus on the depths of The Void, we leave our thoughts, cares, body, and the entire manifest world behind for a time. Those things are not really us, but they're so distracting and feel so "real" in our daily lives that it often feels like they *are* our life.

Our *real life* is the infinite energy and intelligence that hums along quietly inside and keeps us alive, yet we seldom slow down enough to appreciate that which is our purest essence. When you focus on The Void, you experience your pure essence and for all practical purposes go back to the Nothing from which you came and to which you will eventually return. You're free of yourself and everything else—you're completely "out of the way." You know just how out of the way you've gotten when you experience the rested feeling afterward.

You feel the relief in contrast to your former state, which wasn't necessarily bad, but nothing is as resistance-free as The Void, because there is no gravity, no form, no thought there. You naturally want to return to the contrast, gravity, form, and thought of your physical life, because that's what you came here to experience, yet the rest breaks are rejuvenating. You get those rest breaks in sleep, but it's more powerful when it's a conscious choice.

Learn to visit The Void without calling it a meditation, for several reasons. People bring all kinds of baggage to "meditation"—definitions, pre-conceived notions, expectations, a giant toolkit of techniques, past experiences, and beliefs about what it is and what it's supposed to do, and that baggage prevents them from going empty and open—into Nothing, for Nothing.

The small self has a terrible time letting go of all its precious collected stuff. Its worst fear is that it's been wrong. The small self has a tough time saying, "That was true then, but this newer bigger truth will now serve me even better." Poet David Whyte says it beautifully, "In this high place, in this high place, leave everything you know behind."

It's easier to focus on The Void than to try to focus on "nothing." I invite you to experience The Void fresh, from Nothing and as Nothing. "Nothing" is the most pure and potent form (actually non-form) of God, so these visits to the Void take you back home to your Source in the most powerful way.

If there's something you want to solve, never "take that problem to The Void." If the problem is there, you're not in The Void! There are no problems in The Void. Just go there to sit in the powerful stillness and emptiness. That puts you in Large Self state where the problem doesn't exist or is already solved.

Thinking about it gives it energy and reality—
ceasing to think about it diminishes its reality.

You don't need to think, solve, try, or have anything happen during your visits to the Void to get remarkable results in your life. Once you're out of the way, Grace takes over, and ease and magic happen. You let go of the problem, which makes space for a new creation, without working on it.

When you're in the Void, you aren't worrying, stressing, and throwing out limitations or counter-intentions, because you aren't thinking at all. The very acts of scheming and strategizing indicate that you're in the mental vibration, which in story form may sound like, "it's hard" or "I can't let go" or "I have to work at this or figure it out myself." It's amazing what materializes when you just get out of the way and distract yourself from thinking a little bit more often.

Because it's often challenging to hold the new vibration of what we want without contradicting it for long enough to have it appear or occur, it's actually easier to forget about it and get out of the mind altogether.

ACTIVITY: The Fertile Void Meditation

Give yourself a conscious vacation from the denser physical world.

- Sit quietly, smile a tiny smile, and close your eyes.
- Gently focus on your soft breathing, putting every ounce of your attention on your breath.
- Tell yourself to temporarily suspend the formation of words.
- If thoughts arise, don't follow them, let them float away.
- Turn your vision inward and point your attention as if down into your deep interior core. As you keep following that intention deeper into yourself with every breath, you'll eventually come to a restful, quiet, ineffable nothing—the Fertile Void. It is maternal and nurturing and soothing nothing. It feels blissful.
- From this pre-manifest nothing, all things come, and all things return.
- Even spending a few minutes a day in the Void is extraordinarily powerful.

Because The Presence has already created what you want, all that's left for you to do is align with it, or get out of the way, going to the Void for even a few minutes at a time can provide that opportunity for what you want and need to come to you faster and easier. It's another example of working on it less, and getting out of the way more.

Ask or intend once. The Presence has a perfect memory. If it's not happening, you're in the way. Get out of the way. *Of course,* there are actions to take, but first, line up the energy.

You probably won't be able to trace the new developments in your life back to anything specific you did here, because we're not "doing" anything, but you'll know it worked.

Intend the new matrix and forget about it.
Act when you're nudged.

* * * * * * * *

Why Good People Get Hurt

I've joked that spiritual people wouldn't hurt anyone—except themselves. They'll do things that don't feel good, deny themselves pleasure, and put themselves through years of tortuous processing, thinking, "It's good for me." They'll squash their own feelings till they're sick, or put others first until they've drained themselves dry.

When someone pokes a sharp stick in her own eye incessantly, and then screams, "I need a healer!" I'm likely to joke, "You wouldn't if you'd stop poking that stick in your eye."

A woman told me she didn't understand why her marriage fell apart. She talked incessantly about nothing and was completely unaware that her well-meaning, smiley-faced demeanor was pulsing victimhood. In all her stories, she was the good person who always did the right thing and was wronged or under-appreciated.

I counseled her to stop smiling the fake smile, take the emotional hit of the feelings vibrating inside her from the past, and feel her way up the Instrument Panel. She realized she'd been running from feelings her whole life, drowning them with constant babble, and attracting disregard by being a good, spiritual victim. She reclaimed her own power, got genuinely happy, and is a delight to be around. Her blood pressure returned to normal, making medication no longer necessary.

Victims are almost always "good" people, but the "victim" broadcast does not attract goodness, it attracts "villains," just as the smell of blood attracts sharks. Victim vibration is very, very low on the Instrument Panel, and attracts more victimization. One can be powerful and take responsibility for constructing one's own reality, or one can be right and be the good victim, but it's impossible to be both. If you want your power back, say, "I created it," even if you don't know *how* you created it.

When Jesus said, "Turn the other cheek," his disciples erroneously interpreted his words to mean, "Let them hit you again on the other cheek." He meant turn your head away from what you don't want and turn toward what you want. Don't focus attention on what is unwanted. His words could be paraphrased as an admonition to walk away or—I am compelled to bring playfulness to serious subjects—"Turn those *other* cheeks, your backside cheeks to it."

If you've been keeping all your commitments to others but not to yourself, look at this carefully. So many people come to me puzzled that their virtuousness hasn't resulted in more good things happening to *them*. You can't earn power of any kind by being good. Being good doesn't get you extra points with The Presence, because your worthiness was already a given—all you need to do is accept the good you're already offered. It diminishes your power of intention to feel unworthiness, because The Presence does not agree with you.

You can't buy more power of intention by being good. You build your power by being awake, clear, and feeling your worthiness.

Summing it up, people often pulse signals of "victim" or "weak" or "unworthy" when they think they're vibrating "good person."

Power and worthiness aren't given to you.
You just claim them, because they are already yours.

Feel The Fear And Do It Anyway?

"Feel the fear and do it anyway" is one of those clichés that was spawned in the personal development field, and it sounded good, so everyone started parroting it, much to the peril of dare-devils everywhere. Don't get me started on how many misleading myths there are in the metaphysical and spiritual world. Read the free article called "Spiritual Myths That Hold You Back" at DivineOpenings.com. Look in the lower left sidebar under Free Articles.

What are a redneck's famous last words? "Hey, everybody, watch this!" I think Larry The Cable Guy said that.

"Feel the fear and do it anyway" is a monumentally bad piece of advice. When your Instrument Panel reads "trouble," listen to it rather than forging ahead. Align your vibration with your Large Self before taking action. If your airplane's Instrument Panel says you're running out of gas, it would be unwise to feel the fear and keep flying anyway. Land and fuel up.

When you set your intention and then wait until you get the green light to act, you reduce risk. Once you feel good about doing something—when your Instrument Panel has a high reading—your chances of success increase tremendously. If you go into a situation with a low vibration, a low belief level, and a correspondingly low Instrument Panel reading, it's pretty well guaranteed not to turn out like you want it to, no matter how hard you scrunch up your courage, and no matter how strong your intention is.

I'm not saying you can't ever succeed while feeling fear—you can turn some level of fear into productive anger or raw power, but it's a matter of degree, and you can use your Instrument Panel to gauge whether you can make that leap or not. In an emergency, sometimes you have no choice—you must leap, and put yourself in the hands of The Divine. You'll know when to leap.

It's a better bet to take action when your vibration on a subject is high. When it's low, take a break, take a nap, procrastinate just a bit until you get the "go" signal from your inner Presence. But don't allow yourself to stay in resistance for long. Intend to rise out of it.

* * * * * * * *

Intend To Generate Joy

This is going to seem so simple, but all great truths are. One morning recently, I lay in bed reflecting on the interesting phenomenon that in the early stages of Enlightenment you may be blissed out and laugh a lot. I lay there feeling good in a way that ten years ago I could not have imagined, with no worries, no feeling of stress, no problems, in the flow, yet now it just felt... normal. I asked The

Presence Within how to spark that high again, and immediately got the answer as an urge to simply focus on how good it felt to be high—and it all came rushing back. The trees outside my window suddenly looked greener, the air smelled fresher, my body lightened yet more.

How you felt before your awakening began is a big contrast to how you feel right after it begins—it's perhaps the biggest contrast you may ever feel. But you soon get used to any kind of high and it becomes just . . . normal.

For some, the early stages of awakening may feel like their toe is in a light socket, but then that amount of energy becomes normal—and the contrast is never again quite so radical. Our senses perceive contrast more intensely than subtlety or sameness. From other people's perspectives, we might still look like the Energizer Bunny, getting an enormous amount accomplished, radiating joy, and our lives unfolding amazingly well, but to us, it's just . . . normal.

Chasing spiritual highs is something I actually don't recommend (I never do it) because it throws one back into lack and seeking—instead, I suggest deliberately choosing to savor and enjoy daily life by intention. Savor things like lying in bed welcoming the morning, and yes, washing dishes and cleaning house, our modern day versions of chopping wood and carrying water. Remember to express love to people, especially those closest to you.

If I'd lain there lamenting that my old high is now "just normal," I'd have gone lower, because anything we focus upon gets more pronounced. It was fun to experience again the profound truth that what you focus on is what you get.

There's a local taco dive I like to frequent, and one day as I sat there all sweaty after a horseback ride, reading a novel, the owner came over to me and said, "My husband and I see you in here all the time, and you have this… *peace* about you… you radiate… *something*. What do you *do?*"

Initially it was surprising—I thought all I was radiating was sweaty horse smell. I wasn't feeling particularly blissed out. It was an ordinary day for me, but she perceived something out of the ordinary. I said, "I'm a spiritual teacher. I help people get really happy really fast," and gave her my card.

As you build your power of intention, much as when you build a muscle, it gets stronger. Your power of intention works faster, you have "that certain something." You're magnetic and people notice it. Things come to you. Causeless bliss visits.

Focus on the magic and it swells. Remember special times and they return. Evoke the feelings you want more of and they multiply.

> Intend to feel better.
> Intend to feel even better than that while lavishly appreciating how you feel now.
> Intend juicier relationships.
> Intend even juicier relationships while appreciating what you have right now.
> Intend more friendship and love.
> Intend more inner peace.
> Intend even more inner peace while appreciating what you have now.
> Intend deeper inner knowing.
> Intend even deeper inner knowing while appreciating what you have right now and how far you've come.
> Intend greater physical vitality.
> Intend even greater physical vitality while appreciating what you have right now.

Go Where Your Large Self Already Is

More and more you'll simply intend it and it unfolds. You may already be there. Intend in every moment to go where your Large Self is on any topic, to see from your Large Self's perspective, to feel how your Large Self feels about it. It's incredibly simple, yet it automatically expands you and gets you in sync with The Presence.

Your Large Self doesn't have issues, baggage, blocks, blind spots, damage, hurt, limitations, stuck energy, or problems—only endless possibilities in an exuberant, never-ending evolution. This is why issues disappear without working on them with Divine Openings.

Identify with your Large Self, not your problems.

As you live more and more as your Large Self, and experience more deep knowing of your vast Non-Physical resources and power, you simply do not have the issues that a mere human struggling alone in the physical world has. You could work on the small self your whole life or thousands of lives, and it simply would not get fixed. But when you identify as your Large Self, there's *nothing to fix.*

When things in your life aren't like you want them, avoid labeling those things as "issues," even if they've been a problem for a long time. Labeling things as "issues" is using your power of intention to make them into "a big dang official deal." What you really have are simply some thoughts, feelings, and maybe a habitual vibration—which will disappear as you shift your focus to a whole new matrix.

One of the fastest ways to step into infinite possibilities is to identify yourself as your Large Self. Ask Effective Questions to gently move there:

- *How could I perceive this as my Large Self does?*
- *As my Large Self, what is the pulse I emit on this?*
- *As my Non-Physical Self, what possibilities do I hold for this?*
- *How can I get all of me to this party?*
- *How can I celebrate myself more as The Presence in this unique physical human expression?*

Don't answer the questions. Relax and let the answers, inspirations, urges, circumstances, people, or resources appear in the natural course of living. Give yourself some time. Once you experience how good it feels to operate this way, you'll more and more bounce up to Large Self identity automatically.

Lead your mind or it leads you by default!

* * * * * * * *

Direct Knowing

Direct knowing is an advanced capability that can't quite be explained. Information appears in your consciousness, but you don't know how or why you know. You let the information you need flow to you when you need it, and you appreciate it, which causes more of it to flow. You don't have to know how a computer works to be productive with it. You don't have to know how direct knowing works to use it.

If your mind won't let you be happy with "just knowing"—if you must be able to explain it to accept it—you won't fully access your power of direct knowing. You don't have to listen to your mind, however.

I've seen a few people give profound physical healings in the Five Day Silent Retreat, then follow their small self off on a seeking detour trying to figure it out intellectually or "learn how to do" what they already did! Meanwhile the rest of us are giving healings that confound doctors, *without knowing anything*.

When we seek answers outside, and shape our reality around those answers, we give our inner power away. At the very best, we get someone else's version of reality. One of my favorite retorts to well-meaning suggestions to face reality or listen to proven facts is, "That's not *MY* reality, thank you." I've found most of my answers by direct knowing, and have shaped my reality around them. I haven't followed most of the rules of other people's games.

When we're experiencing direct knowing, we gladly give up the false security of proof, logic, and consensus reality. We stop seeking *out there*. That's when we really begin to have fun exploring the possibilities of life, rather than looking for rules, permission, and explanations. We're just happy that it works and that our Non-Physical tech-support team handles all the technical details for us.

We each have a vast Divine Support Team at our service twenty-four hours a day. In the physical plane, humans do have to take action, but our Divine Support Team can do so much of it for us. The possibilities are completely unlimited. Our job is to know we're worthy to call on our team.

Intend to move into direct knowing.

It's fun living in direct knowing, enjoying the automatic download program, in which what you need often appears, independent of experts or texts. You make up your own purpose for living, and you get to decide what you want to do with your life. You're writing your own script rather than asking God or a psychic what your future holds.

I never ask The Presence what I'm supposed to do—there is no *supposed to*. You get to do whatever you like, and The Presence will support you in that. You'll feel inexorably guided and drawn in certain directions, yet completely free to choose. You're one with the world, yet a distinct, unique expression of it. Your direct knowing simply won't submit to linear logic.

Intend to know from within.

You Are That

It's challenging to focus on the Non-Physical until you understand deeply that *there is nothing there!* Having God or guides speak the answer or show us visions are all fine things; sure, The Presence *can* take on a form for you, but that is materialization, not the pure essence of Source. You can directly know and experience Pure Source—that most essential form of God—nothingness, silence, and that feeling of bliss.

Tremendous power, peace, and enjoyment, and yes, even humor come with the deep, *direct experience* of your Large Self. As this knowing of your true Self becomes your new habit, you will look within automatically.

The other day when a friend said, "Thank you, God," before she ate her food, I kept quiet. I'm more inclined toward inner appreciation. There's no separate God "outside" for me to thank. I'm not *all that God is*, but I am God expressing in a physical body and am not separate from God. I giggle at times when I look around and this thought suddenly occurs, "Wow, I'm on this crazy physical planet! Cool!"

More and more, you'll say, "Intend and it is so," rather than "Ask and it is given." Rather than asking, as if God is separate from you, you have the power to intend it. You may not be "all that" but you are that.

You could wait until you leave your physical body to fully know who you are, or you can know now. I'm hearing more and more stories about people lighting up and literally glowing just before they transition out of their bodies. A client's grumpy mother recently became enlightened and lit up in her last days. In the documentary *George Harrison: Living In The Material World* by Martin Scorsese, the former Beatle's wife said although George's spiritual search had been a struggle, he physically illuminated the entire room at his passing. He finally let go.

You'll remember all of who you are at some point—
You might as do it now.

ACTIVITY: Breathe Into The Non-Physical

Your entire reality changes when you begin and end each day focusing on your Non-Physical Self. Sit, smile a tiny smile, and take some slow, deep breaths. Encourage yourself to take a break from forming words. Feel the oxygen permeating every cell in your entire body, bringing expanded consciousness to each cell, waking you up even more. Merge with The Presence. As your power of intention grows, you can simply intend inner focus and you will shift.

* * * * * * * *

Make A Difference In The World
Create A Whole New Matrix

In *Things Are Going Great In My Absence*, you learned how to transition from the old reality of fixing, clearing, and working on things to creating a new reality, from nothing. As you expanded in power, you first noticed that, without trying or saying a word, you had a greater effect on your smaller collectives such as family, friends, community, and workplace. As you become the most powerful component, you can set broad-reaching intentions and have a larger circle of influence.

Practice on personal evolution first and always, and your world fills in to match. Never underestimate the huge difference you make in the world just by being who you are in whatever role you play in life.

Want your world to feel better to you? Right after you feel something you don't like or want to change, drop the old matrix and feel into an entirely new matrix of your choosing. Feel that feeling for just a few minutes and smile. That's all it takes. That pulse ripples out from you, influencing the matrix on every subject: money, relationships, God, society, living on earth, security, etc. Stubbornly stick to it, regardless of the physically materialized product of the old matrix you see in front of you.

Create a new matrix.

Trying to fix the old reality splits your focus between what was and what could be. It's more effective to focus completely on the new matrix. This requires practice until it is a firm habit, and even then requires daily choices.

People who have developed immense power can simply intend evolution for humankind and impact the world. You can call them World Balancers. They're one reason why the world hasn't melted down yet despite all the crazy things we do. Add to them the vast, supportive power of our Divine Support Team, our Non-Physical Selves, the underlying goodness and Grace of life, and the powerful intentions of many humans who preceded us and continue to intend from the Non-Physical, and you can viscerally sense just how big the scope of our power is, including and beyond our human selves.

Of course, you'll notice what's wrong, but to make the biggest difference, bounce off that and focus on the new matrix you want for humanity. You feed energy to whatever you focus on—for better or worse—but when you shift to the new matrix and skip to the payoff, enjoying the feeling of how it will be, you're moving.

For now, each time you want something to change or shift, practice thinking of it this way: you're creating a new matrix, not fixing the old one. Only we hold things in the old forms and patterns. Each day really can be a new day!

Each day can be the product of a new matrix.

Build power, then you can intend larger things. Governments can evolve, for example—it does happen—just not always as fast or precisely as we'd like because it's a collective creation. Co-creations by cultural, social, and political group consciousness often take time to evolve and shift because no single person, including you or me, can control it—it's a shared, collective creation. Each of us can only truly control our own vibration and our own personal reality—but you certainly can create a ripple effect as you think, feel, and pulse a powerful signal. That is how the biggest social change occurs.

Let your new matrix magnetize its own ideal building blocks.

While passion, power, and intention moves mountains (and rocks), attachment always weakens us, whether it's needing a job, an outcome, or a person too much, or getting so specific about how something should play out that we don't allow other, better options in. Be stubbornly committed to the feeling you want, but flexible and unattached to the form it takes. For example, you want the world to be free, but that freedom may or may not look like your own brand of politics. You want our Earth home to be taken care of, but it may or may not look like your version of environmentalism.

Even when we're convinced that a change would be good for someone or even everyone else's own good, imposing our intentions on others is never appropriate. How many religious wars have been fought over what's good for everyone instead of letting each person choose?

Your old matrix is already history, and there's nothing to fix. It's already vaporized unless you keep focusing on it, recreating it, and dragging it on into your next new moment. Be aware of the trap of being right about how wrong the old matrix is—that charge holds you out of the flow. Give no reality and scant attention to the current matrix unless it's what you want more of.

Be a leader, not a sponge.
Be a creator, not a slave to historical fact.

Focus on the long view, the lifetime view, and even the Universal view, just as The Presence does. There's no benefit in letting our vibration plummet because the world is not evolving fast enough, no matter how abhorrent any current reality is—those people are eternal beings and in the cosmic scheme they are alright.

My vibration is my greatest asset. Nothing—nothing—nothing is worth lowering it for long. We can intend, form a new matrix, and go on about our happy life, expecting the best no matter how it looks temporarily.

Some helpful, soothing thoughts and EQ's:

- "I'll focus on how the world is getting better all the time."
- "Visionaries *always* pour their energy into what could be, not what already is."
- "How can I be a steady force for my evolution, and allow that to ripple out naturally?"
- "What intention can I contribute to the world by living it myself?"

Keep most of your daily attention focused on what you are pulsing personally, thus radiating to the collective. As your power increases and as you're able to hold your intention steady and be the most powerful component without getting distracted by the current matrix, you can have a more profound impact on the collective.

At the next level, Jumping The Matrix, you'll move even farther into creating from The Void, from nothing. Remember Neo in the movie *The Matrix* suddenly finding he could not only see the illusion behind the Matrix but dodge bullets as well? While it was unnecessarily "Hollywood" and apocalyptic, parts of that film can help us imagine jumping the current matrix and reclaiming our innate power. Imagination is the seed of change.

First go for deeper and deeper joy and inner power rather than striving for some next level—there is no benefit at all in attaining levels. Many people have told me that they backed off from Jumping The Matrix and went back to Level One or Two when they rushed into it before getting to joy. Fully enjoy where you are now first. Smell the flowers.

Living Into Your Freedom

I clearly intend to set people free, not build a permanent following. If I were to see lots of people still asking me for answers to all their questions after a few years, I'd be disturbed and question the effectiveness of Divine Openings.

Some people do continue to come back for inspiration, connection, and enjoyment of kindred spirits, for an occasional refresher, or to go higher, and that is okay. It's also okay for people to take as long as they need to get free. Everyone is different. Some people actually want a teacher for life. I personally don't—my greatest desire has always been to know from within.

Some people will receive all they need from this book and its predecessor, *Things Are Going Great In My Absence,* while others need more—such as the self-paced online courses, so they can enjoy that vibrational uplift from my live audios and videos, and get live ongoing support on the Member Forum while they practice and create new habits. There is no one-size-fits all plan. Let in all the help you need. This is *your life!*

This is success as I define it: a former student, who also became a friend and someone who would look after my ranch when I was out of town, sent this note along with a gift of some music she thought I would enjoy.

> *I will always love you and be forever grateful for everything I have learned from you. But I know now that my answers lie within me, and I know how to find them. Lots of love to you, Mindy*

My aim is for people who do Divine Openings to be able to go as high as they want, as fast as they are able, and remain stable and functional on planet Earth. I suggest that people go slowly, since there is no rush, grounding their energy step-by-step in their practical life, building a solid foundation, and evolving at a sustainable pace. Bring it down to Earth in your life experience as you expand, unfold, and evolve your own reality—we don't need anyone's permission or validation to do that. We answer our own questions from within or an answer comes to us in some natural way soon after asking, or the question itself simply disappears.

It's a blessed and liberating day when
you just enjoy living and working.

I entered twenty-one days of silence six years ago with a clear intention to end my seeking and go directly to Source, and it happened. I had found out the hard way that I couldn't stop seeking while still seeking, just like you can't stop smoking while still smoking. The best days of my life arrived only after seeking ceased and going exclusively within replaced it.

As deeply committed as I am to helping every student become his or her own master, I constantly endeavor to remain in the background. It's one of the reasons the Internet has been such a uniquely perfect medium to help me serve. I may visit you in dreams or assist you in ways beyond imagining, yet I want no part of guru roles or satsangs, and I try to avoid everything that would lead to others relying on me. Yet some people need or want continuing guidance along the way, and we do offer that in the self-paced online courses, group calls, Member Forum, and live retreats. More and more Divine Openings Givers are offering meetings and events.

My intention is to keep a balance between giving you what you truly need at each stage, and stepping back as you claim your power—reminding you when you need it, and fading back when you remember who you are.

People sometimes have large, unquestioned, unconscious counter-intentions. Some stop at the entrance to the inner cave, intimidated by the imaginary dragon the controlling, fearful mind creates. Some forfeit freedom to stay in the comfort of a group of cherished seeker friends. Some have fears of going direct, and others have that plain old fear of feeling that no amount of seeking can bypass.

At the doorway leading to freedom, chronic followers shrink back into the comfort of the herd and established consensus reality. Yet you are never alone out on the leading edge and the only risk is in not growing—the ultimate connectedness and security is found wholly within you.

Each of you is *the center* of the entire Holographic Universe. Your singular pulsing creates a unique reality, yet you attract many people who experience similar but fascinatingly different realities. When I first moved to Ojai, California, I didn't know a single person here, so, of course, my mind fretted a bit. But less than a year later, I have a weekly date with a friend to ride horses, about ten friends in nearby Los Angeles, and music-making friends close by as well. I'm part of a close-knit group who've been through the Five Day Retreat and we get together to see comedy shows, lounge by the pool at a spa, dine out, and just play. My world has expanded, not shrunk. I've intended that expansion.

Be patient with yourself. It's all okay.

Take a deep breath, sigh it out, and set the intention to relax into the next vibratory level in your own perfect timing—that's right, relax into it, don't work toward it. Allow the power of your intention to expand you without effort.

At each expansion, a door uniquely perfect for you in all the Universe opens, you throw down any remaining crutches, fling your arms wide, and step through the door into the unknown without benefit of definitions, maps, guides, or directions. Without needing anyone to assure or comfort you,

you walk into the new matrix you're creating.

When an engineer imagines a new gadget in his mind and then designs it on the computer, it's essentially Non-Physical. When the physical prototype is built it almost always needs refining. Few inventors produce a physical first prototype that can't be improved upon once it's physical. It's one thing to imagine something into being, and quite another to tweak it until it works.

Whatever you create is a work in progress, and you can tweak it or send it back to The Void for an entirely new design. Floating in the formless, pre-manifest Non-Physical has its value, but physical materialization focuses Energy, Intelligence, and Power in a concentrated way that's vital to the forward march of evolution.

As you test drive your new creations, enjoy the developmental curve rather than lamenting any lack of instant perfection. You have eternity to evolve, and the unfolding is part of the fun.

The material world is a miraculous gift you've given yourself as a place to focus your power and intention, test your creations, and let them unerringly mirror to you what you're vibrating in various areas of your life. Notice that I did not say it's a schoolroom or a proving ground—that's the old paradigm. Instead, see your life as a series of works of art that you're happily never done with, each one more beautiful than the last.

Divine Openings always appreciates and celebrates the material world as the wondrous creation it is. We don't see it as inferior in any way, and certainly not as something to be escaped or transcended. The world is to be mastered, enjoyed, and explored. You came here to experience this wondrous creative workshop.

If you are still skeptical of the claim that the world is getting better all the time, and need something to satisfy your left brain, read *The Rational Optimist*. Author Matt Ridley proves with facts and figures that progress on Earth is indeed on fast-forward, with a recent spike accelerating our evolution to warp speed.

Physicists tell us the Universe is literally expanding. Isn't that metaphorically perfect? We are in constant development, refinement, expansion, and improvement, and our desires for more and better drive evolution. The Universe grows ever bigger because of everything created within it.

Enjoy the procession of moments, many of them mundane, that comprise the real stuff of your life. They're rich and satisfying when you slow down, savor, and fully experience them.

One of my simple daily joys is to wake up and go out to the horse corral and scoop the manure into a neat pile, so the horses don't walk in it. I cannot explain why I take such pleasure in the sun shining on my back, or the fog dampening my coat, the music of birds singing, and the smell of horses and dirt as this daily chore is done. The handy man, thinking he was being gallant, asked me to let him do that chore one day when he was here, and I said, "No, thank you, I love doing this." The corral often looks like a Zen garden when I'm done, with rake marks on the scraped-clean dirt.

When you're willing to fully experience, feel, and embrace it all, this physical space and time is Heaven.

En-joy your life.

* * * * * * * *

Just Intend

Now forget it all and *play with creativity and abandon, with pure intention.* Once you've practiced with each piece this book offers you for a while, you won't have to think about it anymore, just as a tennis pro no longer has to think about her swing because it's become part of her muscle memory.

The experiences in this book aren't meant to load you up with concepts and practices. Ideally, you have read slowly, practiced, formed new habits, and now—you can *relax and intend.*

Remember, at the beginning of the book I told you it's not about what you *do* so much as what *you don't do.* The emptier you are the more you can create from nothing.

Now, you're emptier and you're doing less of these:

- Vibrating counter-intentions
- Leaking power by letting others sit on your throne
- Giving away power by looking outside yourself too much
- Working on yourself
- Giving power to others to fix or heal you
- Letting the physical be your God—focusing too much on the material
- Trying to push rocks up hills with action
- Listening to your mind
- Saying one thing and doing another
- Leaking power in your speech

If you've truly let go, dusted the clutter from your mind, and reclaimed your power, now all there is for you to do anytime you want something is *intend!* No process, no fancy esoteric knowledge—*just intend.* If you feel there's more getting out of the way to do, experience this book again more slowly, and instead of grasping, savor, play, practice, en-joy, and assimilate more. Come back to the book for a refresher if you come up against a new challenge in the future.

Each time you start to throw action at a need or desire,
stop and simply intend it first.

If your intention doesn't materialize, notice how you got in the way and intend for that to shift. So often, all you need to do is intend more clearly and things begin to move in that direction.

For example:

- You want your partner to be more affectionate or prosperous. Intend to give yourself the feelings you'll have with your ideal partner, whether this one or another.

- You want more income. Intend to feel how that feels.
- You'd like a vacation. Intend to generate the feelings of vacation now.
- You'd like your health to improve. Intend it.
- You'd like to lose weight. Intend a lean, light feeling, and then follow through on the nudges you get.
- You'd like to sleep better tonight. Intend it as you go to sleep instead of fretting about not sleeping. You can rest without sleeping and wake energized.

The most beautiful neon-yellow bird, my Dad's favorite color, is trying to peck its way through my window screen a couple of feet away from me as I write—and it has done this before. Hi Dad! Birds offer themselves freely and easily as messengers from the Non-Physical to humans. Writing these words feels so good, and the writing takes me to a place where this bird and my father can connect with me in soaring, freedom, lightness, and joy—the same things he now constantly experiences in the Non-Physical.

The Presence knows your heart's desires better than you know them, and you can indeed let go and let The Divine do the heavy lifting. There is a balance of letting go and deliberately creating—you are not a puppet—you're a powerful Co-Creator who can create intentions and set directions, which The Presence and your Divine Support Team is eager to facilitate for you.

You can combine letting go and setting intentions in this way:
set intention, let go to your Large Self.

The following are some of my own long-term intentions, my all-encompassing lifetime or so-called meta-intentions. I don't work on them, recite them, or even think about them. When we powerfully intend something *once*, the pulse of it radiates out with no effort, unless we get in the way and contradict it. We don't have to hold an intention constantly—our predominant pulse determines our outcomes:

> *Most importantly, I intend to stay awake and live as my Expanded Self.*
>
> *I intend to use my free will daily to make wise and good-feeling choices.*
>
> *I intend to evolve continuously, and by that I uplift humanity.*
>
> *I intend to appreciate and value all feelings.*
>
> *I intend to allow in more of the good that's in my reservoir.*
>
> *I intend to live fully, actively en-joying each day.*
>
> *I intend to keep my body, my vehicle and temporary home, in tip-top condition.*

None of my core intentions are about things—they're about states of being because the most important part of my life is how I feel and flow through life. There is nothing wrong with wanting things—I like things, but they're just a byproduct of how I feel. Materializations show up faster and easier when I focus on the Non-Physical Source of all things rather than on the materializations themselves.

Intentions materialize, and then become permanent elements of your reality. There's no need to express any intention more than once unless you get off track and need to recommit to it. The Presence holds your intention steadily and perfectly. Set intentions anytime, but as you wake up or drift off to sleep, the doors to Non-Physical No-Resistance Land are the most open.

Short-term intentions are just that—they create new matrices that fulfill current desires, and then they become part of your life. Let these starter intentions inspire you to create your own long or short-term intentions:

I intend to unfold and develop my gifts and talents.

I AM a powerful catalyst of human evolution, simply by being my authentic self.

I intend to be there for myself.

I intend to embrace any hurts I feel, and return to my Large Self.

I intend to feel kind, compassionate, and unconditionally loving.

I intend to actively generate love rather than waiting for it to appear.

I intend the pulse I broadcast to feel good to others and me.

I intend to embrace all experiences and feelings, even things I initially resist.

I intend to let resistance do its work, through the contrast and experience life offers, without fretting about it.

I intend to appreciate every bit of expansion as it comes, savor the waiting, and appreciate the gradual, eternal unfolding.

I intend to be the most powerful component in my economy.

I intend to disrespect reality.

I intend a good night's sleep and to wake at 7 a.m.

I intend a fun-loving and peaceful visit with my family.

I intend for to my vocation to feel like vacation.

I intend to assimilate new energies gently.

I intend to en-joy exercise as a treat.

I intend to en-joy nutritious food.

I intend to relax and allow flexibility in my shoulders as I sit at the computer.

I intend increased energy in my body.

I intend to send that incident back to The Void.

Practice setting frequent feeling intentions. Write them in your notebook, and then forget about it.

Dream them up playfully, and then celebrate all successes and feedback.

When you think there's something to work on, fix, or do—stop—tune into your Large Self. Your Large Self is already where you want to be, pulsing that same high, steady broadcast all the time. We wander away at times, but all we have to do is come home.

Start small, intending more and more good feelings, taking score only when it's in your favor, and you'll gain evidence of and confidence in your ability to create higher and higher states of being. As you expand, and things begin to snowball, you'll eventually dare to set intentions you previously felt were unattainable.

We've come full circle from the start of the book:

> Let there be light.

> And there is light.

Now you know that's all there is to it.

Really.

* * * * * * * *

~ The Mantras ~

"The Mantras" was originally conceived as a separate mini-book with illustrations for each powerful and pithy mantra I wanted to share, but I chose to make it a bonus section in this book instead. These mantras are colorful, concise, easy-to-remember touchstones from *Things Are Going Great In My Absence, Watch Where You Point That Thing,* and my sessions and teachings. Use them to train your focus and form powerful new conscious habits.

In "The Mantras Video," which is available at the Divine Openings website, I expand on each mantra to soothe, uplift, entertain you—and even make you laugh—in beautiful natural settings. It can be purchased at DivineOpenings.com/mantras.

Watch where you point that thing.
Aim your mind as deliberately as you would aim a missile—the effect is just as powerful. Energy flows where your attention goes. You literally feed energy to what you focus on.

Intend to transcend.
Your intention alone is enormously powerful. Let it be that easy.

Let your intentions be as light as the touch of a gnat's wing.
Wield power without force.

Don't wait. Generate.
Create the energies and feelings you want *now.*

Rave and appreciate.
Practice until it's a habit.

Soften.
Softening releases resistance instantly.

Attention becomes intention.
You energize what you "pay" attention to.
You're "paying" attention—attention is literally currency.

Say yes.
Saying the word yes sends a signal to your body to make happy chemicals. Say yes to everything you can as soon as you can. Saying yes to things you don't like releases resistance so things can shift. "Here we are—now what?"

Smile.
A small, subtle, intentional smile tells your body you are happy.
It's a short cut to generating higher vibrations.

Make it right.
You might as well. Be willing to discover what's right about whatever occurs.
Embrace all life experience as The Presence does. It's all working *for you* if you let it.

All feelings are good.
Appreciate the information feelings give you. Reclaim the tied-up energy.

Dive in.
Drop the story—feel the feeling.

Don't believe everything you think.
Lead your mind or it leads you by default. The mind is an excellent servant, but a horrific master.

Surf it all.
Surfing is not all crests—there are contrasting troughs, and you have to paddle out to meet the waves. The more you relax and enjoy all of it, the easier it gets.

Wobble till you stabilize.
Love and accept where you are. You might as well—it's where you are.

Focus on the Non-Physical.
The physical world often distracts us from that which is most real and powerful.

Bring all of you to the party.
Your Non-Physical Self has started your party. Now get yourself there.

Stay awake.
It's a daily choice.

Worthiness is a given.
It's already yours, and it's there waiting for you to claim or declare it.

It's temporary.
Everything is temporary—remind yourself of that if you don't like what is.

Feelings are actual manifestations to celebrate.
Feeling better is everything. Sure, it's predictive of things that will materialize, but to feel good is why you wanted it to materialize in the first place.

Forget the form.
Focus on the feeling you want and let The Presence bring you the best form.

Skip to the payoff.
Experience what you want as if it's already here and you get to feel the good feelings *now*.

Recognize your Oneness with what you want.
You are never separate from anyone or anything.

Savor the waiting.
Enjoy the dreaming of it and the coming of it as much as the having of it and you feel good now.

Intend, SMILE, and let go.

That's all there is to it.

Visualize just for pleasure.
You don't need to visualize to create it—it's already created. Visualize to feel good now.

It's in your reservoir.
It's already created. It's already yours. Relax.

It's feedback, not failure.
Drop the story. Everything brings forward movement unless we resist. You can't lose and you can't go backwards. Aim, fire, re-aim. Aim, fire, re-aim.

I created that.
I'm making it all up.

Don't take score if it's not in your favor.
Cheat. Because it feels better, only take score of what's good and what's working.

Bounce off the bottom.
Use that resistance in your favor. Stay rubberized.

Each wave is a new wave.
You always get another chance. History doesn't repeat unless we hold onto that vibration.

Slower is faster.
Relaxing into the flow gets it done faster than rushing and stressing.

Resistance is your friend.
Don't resist your resistance. That just adds resistance to resistance. Make resistance Okay and let it work for you.

Contrast is your friend.
What you don't want clarifies what you do want. Contrast isn't always something you don't want—sometimes it's just a matter of choices and which feels better to you, like chocolate and vanilla are contrasts.

If it's too big for you, give it over.
Challenge is fun, but when it's too much, give it over. If you take it back, give it over again.

Learn to drive.
You're a co-creator with The Presence. Take the wheel and drive.

You don't have to know how it works.
Intellectual understanding is the booby prize.

Be the most powerful component.
The most powerful component in an interaction prevails.

En-joy it.
You put the joy into it.

Don't worship the gift.
Cherish and focus on the Giver.
Gifts come and go, but the Giver is eternal and always there for you.

Balance your inner Non-physical and your outer physical life.
Live life in this world in continual awareness of its Source.

You're either a Sponge or a Leader.
You can't be both. Lead with the vibration of how you want things to be, whether people approve or not, whether they come along with you or not.

Your power is now.
The magic date is today. The power is in you. The power spot is where you are.

Sit on the Throne Of Your Own Life.
Kick everyone else off. They have their own throne.

Family—my job is to love them, not to change them.
Period.

Effective Questions open new possibilities.
How does my Large Self experience this? What more is possible?

Go to Large Self Perspective.
It instantly looks and feels better.

Make a preset on your radio dial for Large Self vibration.
The more you go there the more automatic it gets.

Keep your own counsel.
Chat with The Presence often. Take needs and questions inside first.

Lighten up rather than tighten up.
Remind yourself you're making it all up, and that it always works out.

Make the most of the best and the least of the worst.
Your attitude towards it creates how it goes.

Movement is more important than arrival or perfection.
Notice how far you've come, and continue to celebrate your smallest movement.

It's not about having it all right now.
It's about enjoying each new expansion.

Stop pushing rocks up hills.
Let The Divine do the heavy lifting. Focus on what you want.

Chunk it down.
Small, steady steps add up to big results.

Do your High Payoff Activities first.
It's not how much you're doing, it's how much you're doing the right things.

Cut work to a fraction.
Align energy first, then take action. Don't do too much, but do something.

Don't take action when there's an alien on your face.
Wait until you're feeling good to make big plans or decisions or talk about sensitive things.

Line it up. Let it go. Let it in.
Align the energy, release all attachments to the outcome, and soften.

Get in alignment first.
Energy alignment first, action as guided.

Talk is never casual—it's causal.
Words have power. Use them wisely.

And from my former assistant, Crystal:
"It's my rodeo and everybody else is just ridin' in it."

ADDITIONAL RESOURCES:

ONLINE SELF-PACED RETREATS

The Level One Online Retreat helps people stabilize in their new reality during or after reading the foundational book *Things Are Going Great In My Absence*.

The Level Two Online Retreat contains completely new and original material beyond *Things Are Going Great In My Absence* and Level One. Level Two Online is the comprehensive guide to creating a joyful life beyond suffering and problem focus, and it supports you in applying this book.

Level Three, Jumping The Matrix, helps you reach beyond this reality. The courses must be taken in order, as each builds upon the previous ones. Each of my many courses takes you into completely new territory, introduces entirely new material, and introduces next level energies. In this book, we touch only lightly on the energies of Level Three, Jumping The Matrix. Perhaps one day I'll write a Jumping The Matrix book to go with the online course. That course, comprised of twenty-six long, in-depth modules, is already as packed with new material as a complete book. Even if you've completed Level Two, Jumping The Matrix is best done after you've attained relative stability in your life and emotions—powerfully altering your reality always brings an element of destabilization.

First Aid for Special Topics helps people who are in crisis in an area of their lives.

The Art Of Love And Sex Tantric Online Retreat

The Divine Healing Course, with Cathy Ulrich

VIDEOS AND AUDIOS

Each online course includes an extensive library of audios and videos.

Others like these are purchased separately:

The Mantras Video at DivineOpenings.com/mantras

Session audios, original music videos, see DivineOpenings.com menu

LIVE RETREATS

Five-Day Silent Retreats

One-Day Retreats

OTHER BOOKS BY LOLA JONES

Things Are Going Great In My Absence: How To Let Go And Let The Divine Do The Heavy Lifting

Dating To Change Your Life

Divine Openings Quotes

Confessions Of A Cowgirl Guru, coming soon

MUSIC BY LOLA JONES

Watch Where You Point That Thing – twelve songs on CD, including the original song from the film *Beautiful Faces.*

"Here In My Heart"

"Lola's Gayatri Mantra"

"Lolabye"

"Starlight"

All are downloadable at DivineOpenings.com

ART BY LOLA JONES

See DivineOpenings.com

CPSIA information can be obtained at www.ICGtesting.com
Printed in the USA
LVOW091515100513

333274LV00001B/40/P